THE BLACK D

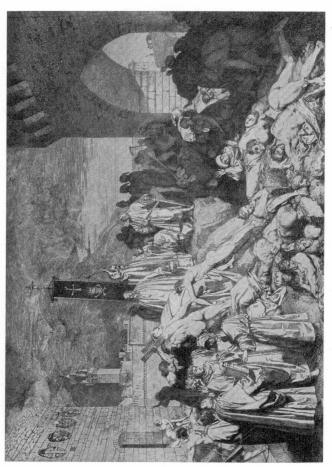

"The Plague of Florence, described by Boccaccio"
by Luigi Sabatelli, 1801

THE BLACK DEATH
A CHRONICLE OF THE PLAGUE

COMPILED BY

JOHANNES NOHL

FROM CONTEMPORARY SOURCES

TRANSLATED BY
C. H. CLARKE

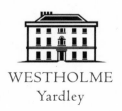

WESTHOLME
Yardley

Originally Published in 1926 by George Allen & Unwin Ltd.
First Westholme Paperback 2006
New material © 2006 Westholme Publishing

Published by Westholme Publishing, LLC
Eight Harvey Avenue, Yardley, Pennsylvania 19067

ISBN 10: 1-59416-029-5
ISBN 13: 978-1-59416-029-5

www.westholmepublishing.com

Printed in United States of America

PREFACE

THIS book is an attempt to depict the plague in its entirety, with all its social consequences. A comprehensive cultural study of this nature has as yet not been published. Georg Sticker, doubtless the greatest authority on this subject, in his excellent two-volume treatise on the Plague, addresses in the first instance the Medical Profession. Interesting as it would have been on the basis of his research to produce evidence of the numerous exact and excellent observations underlying the apparently nonsensical assertions of old-time plague authorities, I have, in order to preserve the uniform character of treatment, refrained from so doing. The purpose of my work is in the first instance to demonstrate the devastating inroads made in former times by epidemics into the spiritual and social life of the various nations. At the hands of historians the effects of the plague have not received a just appreciation. Barthold Georg Niebuhr, who in 1816 wrote as follows, forms an exception :

" The plague not only depopulates and kills, it gnaws the moral stamina and frequently destroys it entirely ; thus the sudden demoralisation of Roman society from the period of Mark Antony may be explained by the Oriental plague—as 600 years before the epidemic, which was really of the nature of yellow fever, coincided too exactly with the decay of the best period of antiquity not to be regarded as its cause. In such epidemics the best were invariably carried off and the survivors deteriorated morally.

" Times of plague are always those in which the bestial and diabolical side of human nature gains the upper hand. Nor is it necessary to be superstitious or even pious to look upon great plagues as a conflict of the terrestrial forces with the development of mankind ; I fear that my conviction of the victory of the negative, destructive forces in this struggle may strike many as by far too Manichæan and godless."

THE BLACK DEATH

Of more modern authors I have referred particularly to the following: J. F. E. Hecker ("The Black Death in the Fourteenth Century," Berlin, 1832), Georg Sticker ("The Plague," Giessen, 1908–1910), Wilhelm Sahm ("History of the Plague in East Prussia," Leipzig, 1905), Hermann Schoeppler ("History of the Plague at Regensburg," 1914), Heino Pfannenschmidt ("Contribution to the History of the German and Dutch Flagellants," Leipzig, 1900), Paul Runge ("Songs of the Flagellants," 1900), Paul Gaffarel et Marquis de Durant ("*La Peste de 1720 à Marseille*," Paris, 1911).

The translation of the Flagellant Chronicle of Hugo of Reutlingen by State Councillor Renaud of Colmar is reproduced from the work of Paul Runge.

JOHANNES NOHL.

Berlin,
Autumn of 1924.

CONTENTS

ILLUSTRATIONS

PLATES
(FOLLOWING PAGE 160)

ILLUSTRATIONS IN THE TEXT

THE BLACK DEATH

CHAPTER I

THE ASPECT OF THE PLAGUE

The deadly galleys—Visitation of Messina—The progress of death—Boccaccio's narrative—Symptoms and course of the plague—Infected animals—Lack of charity—Epitaphs—Death dances—Celebrated victims of the plague—Number of deaths during " Black Death."

Appendices : Letter from Naples—Letter from Danzic—Circumstantial narrative by Abraham a Santa-Clara.

"O HAPPY posterity, who will not experience such abysmal woe and will look upon our testimony as a fable." With these words Petrarch concludes his well-known letter in which he describes to a friend the devastation of the town of Florence by the " Black Death." In the years 1345 to 1350 half the population, or, as is maintained by others, one-third of the population, had succumbed to the plague. Two hundred thousand market towns and villages in Europe were completely depopulated, and in the dwellings encumbered with corpses wild beasts took up their abode. Statistics drawn up at the instigation of Pope Clement VI state the number of deaths for the whole world at 42,836,486.

The name " Black Death," which was commonly given to the plague of 1348, must be regarded as the expression of the horror aroused by this uncanny disease. Popular imagination depicted it as a man mounted on a black horse, or else as a black giant striding along, his head reaching above the roofs of the houses.

The origin of the plague lay in China, and there it is said to have commenced to rage already in the year 1333, after a terrible mist emitting a fearful stench and infecting the air.

From China it passed via India, Persia, and Russia by means
of the three main arteries of commerce then existing to
Europe. The Franciscan friar, Michael of Piazza, describes
its arrival in Sicily: " At the beginning of October, in the
year of the incarnation of the Son of God 1347, twelve Genoese
galleys were fleeing from the vengeance which our Lord was
taking on account of their nefarious deeds and entered the
harbour of Messina. In their bones they bore so virulent a
disease that anyone who only spoke to them was seized by
a mortal illness and in no manner could evade death. The
infection spread to everyone who had any intercourse with
the diseased. Those infected felt themselves penetrated by
a pain throughout their whole bodies and, so to say, under-
mined. Then there developed on their thighs or on their
upper arms a boil about the size of a lentil which the people
called ' burn boil' (antrachi). This infected the whole body,
and penetrated it so that the patient violently vomited blood.
This vomiting of blood continued without intermission for
three days, there being no means of healing it, and then the
patient expired. But not only all those who had intercourse
with them died, but also those who had touched or used any
of their things. When the inhabitants of Messina discovered
that this sudden death emanated from the Genoese ships they
hurriedly expulsed them from their harbour and town. But
the evil remained with them and caused a fearful outbreak of
death. Soon men hated each other so much that, if a son
was attacked by the disease, his father would not tend him.
If, in spite of all, he dared to approach him, he was immediately
infected and could by no means escape death, but was bound
to expire within three days. Nor was this all : all those
belonging to him, dwelling in the same house with him, even
the cats and other domestic animals, followed him in death.
As the number of deaths increased in Messina many desired
to confess their sins to the priests and to draw up their last
will and testament. But ecclesiastics, lawyers and attorneys
refused to enter the houses of the diseased. But if one or the
other had set foot in such a house to draw up a will or for
any other purpose, he was hopelessly abandoned to sudden
death. Minor friars and Dominicans and members of other
orders who heard the confessions of the dying were themselves

immediately overcome by death, so that some even remained in the rooms of the dying. Soon the corpses were lying forsaken in the houses. No ecclesiastic, no son, no father and no relation dared to enter, but they paid hired servants with high wages to bury the dead. But the houses of the deceased remained open with all their valuables, with gold and jewels ; anyone who chose to enter met with no impediment, for the plague raged with such vehemence that soon there was a shortage of servants and finally none at all. When the catastrophe had reached its climax the Messinians resolved to emigrate. One portion of them settled in the vineyards and fields, but a larger portion sought refuge in the town of Catania, trusting that the holy virgin Agatha of Catania would deliver them from their evil. To this town the Queen of Sicily came and summoned her son Don Federigo. In November the Messinians persuaded the Patriarch, Archbishop of Catania, to permit the relics of the saints to be brought to their town. But the populace of Catania would not allow the sacred bones to be removed from their old place. Now intercessary processions and pilgrimages were undertaken to Catania to propitiate God. But the plague raged with greater vehemence than before. Flight was no longer of avail. The disease clung to the fugitives and accompanied them everywhere where they turned in search of help. Many of the fleeing fell down by the roadside and dragged themselves into the fields and bushes to expire. Those who reached Catania breathed their last in the hospitals there. The terrified citizens demanded from the Patriarch prohibition on pain of ecclesiastical ban, of burying fugitives from Messina within the town, and so they were all thrown into deep trenches outside the walls.

" The population of Catania was so godless and timid that no one among them would have intercourse or speak to the fugitives, but each hastily fled on their approach. But if some fugitive wished to address them they said : ' Do not speak to me, you are from Messina ! ' And no one offered them shelter. If some relations in Catania had not secretly harboured a number of people from Messina, they would have been deprived of all assistance. Thus the people of Messina dispersed over the whole island of Sicily and came also to

Syracuse and with them the disease, so that in Syracuse innumerable people died. Sciacca, Trapani, Girgenti, and Messane, thus, were also infected by the plague, but particularly Trapani, which was completely depopulated. The town of Catania lost all its inhabitants, so that it ultimately sank into complete oblivion. Here not only the ' burn blisters ' appeared, but there developed in different parts of the body gland boils in some on the sexual organs, in others on the thighs, in others on the arms, and in others on the neck. At first these were of the size of a hazel-nut and developed accompanied by violent shivering fits, which soon rendered those attacked so weak that they could no longer stand upright, but were forced to lie in their beds consumed by violent fever and overcome by great tribulation. Soon the boils grew to the size of a walnut, then to that of a hen's egg or a goose's egg, and they were exceedingly painful, and irritated the body, causing it to vomit blood by vitiating the juices. The blood rose from the affected lungs to the throat, producing on the whole body a putrifying and ultimately decomposing effect. The sickness lasted three days, and on the fourth, at the latest, the patient succumbed. As soon as anyone in Catania was seized with headache and shivering, he knew that he was bound to pass away within the specified time, and first confessed his sins to the priest and then made his last will. When the plague had attained its height in Catania, the Patriarch endowed all ecclesiastics, even the youngest, with all priestly powers for the absolution of sin which he himself possessed as bishop and patriarch. But the pestilence raged from October 1347 to April 1348. The Patriarch himself was one of the last to be carried off. He died fulfilling his duty. At the same time Duke Giovanni, who had carefully avoided every infected house and every patient, died."

Two freight-ships then carried the disease from Messina to Pisa. The crews of both the ships were suffering from the plague, and all those in Pisa who spoke to the sailors on Piazza dei Pesci were seized and died immediately. This was in the first days of the year 1348. " And thereupon," the chronicle writer Sercambi continues, " there began a great dying in Pisa, and from there spread over the whole of Tuscany. And it raged most fearfully at Lucca. During this great epidemic

of death there died of an hundred more than eighty, and the
air was so infested that death overtook men everywhere,
wherever they might flee. And when they saw everybody
dying they no longer heeded death and believed that the end
of the world was at hand."

That the Province of Tuscany was the first to be assailed
by the plague may be explained by the close commercial
relations which existed, particularly between it and the whole
Neapolitan coast. On the outbreak of the plague in Florence,
and the triumphs it achieved there from April till September,
we possess the classical description of Giovanni Boccaccio,
whose father was carried off by the plague in 1348. The
renowned plague descriptions by the ancient poets and historians—I refer to Ovid, Seneca, Thucydides, Lucrece, Lucan
—served as models for the poet, and yet he has surpassed them
all in vigour and vividness of colouring.

¹ " The yeare of our blessed Saviours incarnation, 1348,
that memorable mortality happened in the excellent City, farre
beyond all the rest in Italy ; which plague, by operation of
the superiour bodies, or rather for our enormous iniquities,
by the just anger of God was sent upon us mortals. Some
few yeeres before, it tooke beginning in the Easterne partes,
sweeping thence an innumerable quantity of living soules :
extending itselfe afterward from place to place Westward,
untill it seized on the said City. Where neither humane skill
or providence, could use any prevention, notwithstanding it
was cleansed of many annoyances, by dilligent officers thereto
deputed : besides prohibition of all sickly persons entrance
and all possible provision dayly used for the conservation of
such as were in health, with incessant prayers and supplications
of devoute people, for the asswaging of so dangerous a sicknesse.

"About the beginning of the yeare it also began in very
strange manner, as appeared by divers admirable effects ;
yet not as it had done in the East Countries, where Lord or

¹ The translation of Boccaccio's description of the plague of 1348 at
Florence is taken from : The Modell/of Wit, Mirth, Eloquence/and Conver-
sation/framed in ten dayes, of an hundred/curious pieces, by seven Honour-
able/Ladies, and three Noble Gentlemen/preserved to posterity by the
renowned/John Boccaccio/The first Refiner of Italian Prose/and now translated into English./1625./ (Translator not known.)

Lady being touched therewith, manifest signes of inevitable death, followed thereon, by bleeding at the nose. But there it began with yong children, male and female, either under the armpits, or in the groine by certaine swellings, in some to the bignesse of an Apple, in others like an Egge, and so in divers greater or lesser, which (in their vulgar Language) they termed to be a Botch or Byle. In very short time after, those two infected parts were growne mortiferous, and would disperse abroad indifferently, to all parts of the body ; whereupon, such was the quality of the disease, to shew itselfe by black or blew spottes, which would appeare on the armes of many, others on their thighes, and every part else of the body : in some great and few, in others small and thicke.

"Now, as the Byle (at the beginning) was an assured sign of neere approaching death ; so proved the spots likewise to such as had them : for the curing of which sicknesse it seemed, that the Physitians counsell, the vertue of Medicines, or any application else, could not yield any remedy : but rather it planely appeared, that either the nature of the disease would not endure it, or ignorance in the Physitians could not comprehend from whence the cause proceeded, and so by consequent, no resolution was to be determined. Moreover beside the number of such as were skilfull in Art, many more both women and men, without ever having any knowledge in Physicke, became Physitians : so that not onely few were healed, but (wellneere) all dyed, within three days after the saide signs were seene ; some sooner, and others later, commonly without either Feaver, or any other accident.

"And this pestilence was yet of farre greater power or violence ; for, not onely healthfull persons speaking to the sicke, coming to see them, or ayring cloathes in kindnesse to comfort them, was an occasion of ensuing death : but touching their garments, or any foode whereon the sick person fed, or any thing else used in his service, seemed to transferre the disease from the sicke to the sound, in very rare and miraculous manner. Among which matter of marvel let me tell you one thing, which if the eyes of many (as well as mine owne) had not seene, hardly could I be perswaded to write it, much lesse to beleeve it, albeit a man of good credit should report it. I say, that the quality of this contagious pestilence was not onely of such efficacy, in taking and catching it one of another, either men or women : but it extended further, even in the apparent view of many, that the cloathes, or any thing else, wherein one died of that disease, being toucht, or lyen on by any beast, farre from the kind or quality of man, they did not onely contaminate and infect the said beast, were it Dogge, Cat, or any other ; but also it died very soone.

" Mine owne eyes (as formerly I have said) among divers others, one day had evident experience heereof : for some poor ragged cloathes of linnen and wollen, torn from a wretched body dead of that disease, and hurled in the open streete ; two Swine going by, and (according to their naturall inclination) seeking for foode on every dung-hill, tossed and tumbled the cloathes with their snouts, rubbing their heads likewise upon them ; and immediately, each turning twice or thrice about, they both fell down dead on the saide cloathes, as being fully infected with the contagion of them : which accident, and other the like, if not far greater, begat divers feares and imaginations in them that beheld them, all tending to a most inhumane and uncharitable end ; namely, to flie thence hence from the sicke, and touching any thing of theirs by which means they thought their health should be safely warranted.

" Some there were who considered with themselves, that living soberly, with abstinence from all superfluity ; it would be sufficient resistance against all hurtfull accidents. So combining themselves in a sociable manner, they lived as separatists from all other company, being shut up in such houses, where no sicke body should be neere them. And there, for their more security, they used delicate viands and excellent wines, avoiding luxurie, and refusing speech to one another, not looking forth at the windowes, to heare no cries of dying people, or see any coarses carried to buriall ; but having musicall instruments, lived there in all possible pleasure. Others, were of a contrary opinion, who avouched, that there was no other physicke more certaine, for a disease so desparate, than to drinke hard, be merry among themselves, singing continually, walking everywhere, and satisfying their appetites with whatever they desired, laughing and mocking at every mournful accident, and so they vowed to spend day and night : for now they would go to one Taverne, then to another, living

without any rule or measure ; which they might very easily
doe, because every one of them (as if he were to live no longer
in this World) had even forsaken all things that hee had
By meanes whereof, the most part of the houses were become
common, and all strangers might do the like (if they pleased
to adventure it) even as boldly as the Lord or owner, without
any let or contradiction.

"Yet in all this their beastly behaviour, they were wise
enough to shun (so much as they might) the weake and sickly.
In misery and affliction of our City, the venerable authority
of the Lawes, as well divine as humane, was even destroyed,
as it were through want of lawfull Ministers of them. For
they being all dead, or lying sicke with the rest, or else lived
so solitary, in such great necessity of servants and attendants,
as they could not execute any office, whereby it was lawfull
for every one to do as he listed.

" Between these two rehearsed extremities of life, there
were other of a more moderate temper, not being so daintily
dieted as the first, nor drinking so dissolutely as the second ;
but used all things sufficient for their appetites, and without
shutting up themselves walked abroad, some carrying sweete
nose-gayes of flowers in their hands ; others odoriferous herbes,
and others divers kinds of spiceries, holding them to their
noses, and thinking them most comfortable for the braine,
because the ayre seemed to be much infected by the noysome
smell of dead carkases, and other hurtfull savours. Some
other there were also of more inhumane mind (howbeit per-
adventure it might be the surest) saying, that there was no
better physicke against the pestilence, nor yet so good, as to
flie away from it, which argument mainely moving them, and
caring for no body but themselves, very many both men and
women, forsooke the City, their owne houses, their Parents,
Kindred, Friends, and Goods, flying to other mens dwellings
else-where. As if the wrath of God, in punishing the sinnes
of men with the plague, would fall heavily upon none, but
such as were enclosed within the City wals ; or else perswading
themselves, that not any should there bee left alive, but that
the finall ending of all things was come.

" Now albeit these persons in their diversity of opinions
died not all, so undoubtedly they did not all escape ; but many

among them becoming sicke, and making a general example
of their flight and folly, among them that could not stirre out
of their beds, they languished more perplexedly than the
other did. Let us omit that one Citizen fled after another,
and one neighbour had not any care of another, Parents nor
kinred ever visiting them, but utterly they were forsaken on
all sides : this tribulation pierced into the hearts of men, and
with such a dreadfull terrour, that one Brother forsooke
another, the Unkle the Nephew, the Sister the Brother, and
the Wife the Husband : nay, a matter much greater, and
almost incredible ; Fathers and Mothers fled away from their
owne Children, even as if they no way appertained to them.
In regard whereof, it could be no otherwise, but that a
countlesse multitude of men and women fell sicke ; finding
no charity among their friends, except a very few, and subject
to the avarice of servants, who attended them constrainedly
(for great and unreasonable wages) yet few of these attendants
to be found any where too. And they were men and women
but of base condition, as also of groser understanding, who
never before had served in any such necessities, nor indeed
were any way else to be imployed ; but to give the sicke person
such things as he called for, or to awaite the houre of his
death ; in the performance of which service, oftentimes for
gaine, they lost their owne lives.

" In this extreme calamity, the sicke being thus forsaken of
neighbors, kinred, and friends, standing also in such need
of servants ; a custome came up among them, never heard
of before, that there was not any woman, how noble, young,
or faire soever she was, but falling sicke, she must of necessity
have a man to attend her, were hee young or otherwise, respect
of shame or modesty no way prevailing, but all parts of her
body must be discovered to him, which (in the like urgency)
was not to be seen by any but women : whereon ensued
afterward, that upon the parties healing and recovering, it
was the occasion of further dishonesty, which many being
more modestly curious of, refused such disgracefull attending,
chusing rather to die, than by such helpe to bee healed. In
regard whereof, as well as through the want of convenient
remedies (which the rich by no meanes could attaine unto)
as also the violence of the contagion, the multitude of them

that died night and day, was so great, that it was a dreadfull sight to behold, and as much to heare spoken of So that meere necessity (among them that remained living) begat new behaviours, quite contrary to all which had beene in former times, and frequently used among the City Inhabitants.

"The custome of precedent days (as now againe it is) was that women, kinred, neighbours, and friends, would meete together at the deceased parties house, and there with them that were of neerest alliance, expresse their hearts sorrow for their friends losse. If not thus they would assemble before the doore, with many of the best Cittizens and kindred, and (according to the quality of the deceased) the Cleargy met there likewise, and the dead body was carried (in comely manner) on mens shoulders, with funerall pompe of Torch light, and singing, to the Church appointed by the deceased. But these seemely orders, after that the fury of the pestilence began to encrease, they in like manner altogether ceased, and other new customes came in their place ; because, not onely people died without having any women about them, but infinities also past out of this life, not having any witnesse, how, when, or in what manner they departed. So that few or none there were to deliver outward show of sorrow and grieving : but instead thereof, divers declared idle joy and rejoycing, a use soone learned of immodest women, having put off all feminine compassion, yea, or regard for their owne welfare.

"Very few also would accompany the body to the grave, and they not any of the Neighbours, although it had beene an honourable Citizen, but onely the meanest kinde of people, such as were grave-makers, coffin-bearers, or the like, that did these services onely for money, and the beere being mounted on their shoulders, in all hast they would runne away with it, not perhaps to the Church appointed by the dead, but to the neerest at hand, having some foure or sixe poore Priests following with lights or no lights, and those of the silliest ; short service being said at the buriall, and the body unreverently being throwne into the first open grave they found. Such was the pittifull misery of poore people, and divers, who were of better condition, as it was most lamentable to behold ; because the greater number of them, under hope of healing, or compelled by poverty, kept still within their house weake and faint, thousands falling sicke daily, and having no helpe or being succoured any way with foode or physicke, all of them died, few or none escaping.

"Great store there were, that died in the streetes by day or night, and many more beside, although they died in their houses; yet first they made it knowne to their neighbours, that their lives perished, rather by the noysome smell of dead and putrified bodies, then by any violence of the disease in themselves So that of these and the rest, dying in this manner every where, the neighbours observed one course of behaviour, (moved thereto no less by feare, that the smell and corruption of dead bodies should harme them, then charitable respect of the dead) that themselves when they could, or being assisted by some bearers of coarses, when they were able to procure them, would hale the bodies (already dead) out of their houses, laying them before their doores, where such as passed by, especially in the mornings, might see them lying in no meane numbers. Afterward, Bieres were brought thither, and such as might not have the helpe of Bieres, were glad to lay them on tables, and Bieres have bin observed, not onely to be charged with two or three dead bodies at once, but many times it was seene also, that the wife with the husband, two or three Brethren together ; yea, the Father and the Mother, have thus beene carried along to the grave upon one Biere.

"Moreover, oftentimes, it hath beene seene, that when two Priests went with one Crosse to fetch the body ; there would follow (behind) there or four bearers with their Bieres, and when the Priests intended the burriall but of one body, sixe or eight more have made up the advantage, and yet none of them being attended by any seemly company, lights, teares, or the very least decencie, but it plainly appeared, that the very like account was then made of Men or Women, as if they had bene Dogges or Swine. Wherein might manifestly bee noted, that that which the naturall course of things could not shew to the wise, with rare and little losse to wit, the patient support of miseries and misfortunes, even in their greatest height : not onely the wise might now learne, but also the very simplest people ; and in such sort, that they should alwaies bee prepared against all infelicities whatsoever.

"Hallowed ground could not now suffice, for the great multitude of dead bodies which were daily brought to every Church in the City, and every houre in the day ; neither could the bodies have proper place of buriall, according to our ancient custome : wherefore, after that the Churches and Church-yards were filled, they were constrained to make use of great deepe ditches, wherein they were buried by hundreds at once, ranking dead bodies along in graves, as Merchandizes are laide along in ships, covering each after other with a small quantity of earth, and so they filled at last up the whole ditch to the brim.

"Now, because I would wander no further in everie particularity, concerning the miseries happening in our Citie : I tell you that extremities running on in such manner as you have heard, little lesse spare was made in the Villages round about ; wherein (setting aside enclosed Castles which were now filled like to small Cities) poore Labourers and Husbandmen, with their whole Families, dyed most miserably in out-houses, yea in the open fields also ; without any assistance of physicke, or helpe of servants ; and likewise in the highwayes, or their ploughed landes, by day or night indifferently, yet not as men, but like brute beasts.

"By means whereof, they became lazie and slothfull in their dayly endeavours, even like to our Citizens ; not minding or medling with their wonted affaires, but as a waiting for death every houre, imployed all their paines, not in caring any way for themselves, their cattle, or gathering the fruits of the earth, or any of their accustomed labours ; but rather wasted and consumed even such as were for their instant sustenance. Whereupon it fell so out, that their Oxen, Asses, Sheepe and Goates, their Swine, Pullen, yea their verie Dogges, the truest and faithfullest servants to men, being beaten and banished from their houses, went wildly wandering abroad the fields, where the Corne grew still on the ground without gathering, or being so much as reapt or cut. Many of the foresaid beasts (as endued with reason) after they have pastured themselves in the day time would returne full fed at night home to their houses, without any Government of Heardsmen or any other.

"How many faire Palaces ! How many goodly Houses ! How many noble habitations, filled before with families of

Lords and Ladies, were then to be seene emptie, without any
one there dwelling, except some silly servant ? How many
Kindreds worthy of memory ! How many great inheritances !
And what plenty of riches ; were left without any true suc-
cessours ? How many good men ! How many worthy Women !
How many valiant and comely young men, whom none but
Galen, Hippocrates and Æsculapius (if they were living) could
have been reputed any way unheathfull ; were seene to
dine at morning with their Parents, Friends and familiar

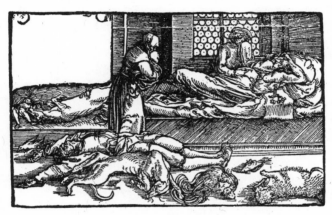

THE PLAGUE IN THE HOMESTEAD.
Woodcut by Hans Weiditz.

confederates and went to sup in another world with their
Predecessors ? ''

Concerning the form in which the plague developed in
Europe there are varying reports. A Thuringian chronicle
thus reports : " Those who were infected by the pestilential
poison lay asleep for three days and nights and, when they
awoke, they immediately began to struggle with death, until
they gave up the ghost." During the plague in Austria in
the year 1679 the sick are said to have succumbed within
twenty-four hours. That animals were also subject to infection is reported by the majority of chronicle writers. Dogs
and cats died, horses, oxen, goats and sheep grew mangy,

wasted away and died within a few days. It is reported that
even the wolves fled at the approach of the grazing cattle
of the farmers. A fact reported from Vienna is worthy of
mention. The physicians during the month of April, in hot
weather, tested the danger to be feared from the quantity
of corpses. They hanged up a dog above a trench in which
some thousand people were lying buried. When after three
hours the dog had ceased to live, they concluded that more
earth should be heaped on the trench.

The most terrible consequence of the danger of infection
was that the patients were forsaken by everyone, even by
their nearest relations. "Then there was no love, no faithfulness, no trust. No neighbour would lend a helping hand
to another. One brother had forsaken the other, husbands
had forsaken their wives, wives their husbands, parents their
children, children their parents. The people died not only of
the plague, but from all kinds of want and privation."

A German poem of the seventeenth century says :

> What misery prevaileth now ?
> In all the streets throughout the land
> The houses now forsaken stand,
> And fathers children leave to die,
> And children from their parents fly,
> And no man hastens at the call
> Of those that stricken downward fall.

"The patient lay helpless and forsaken in his dwelling,
no relation came near him, at the most his best friends were
huddled up in some corner. The physician did not dare to
visit him, the terrified priest trembling offered the Sacraments
of the Church. With heart-rending supplication children called
for their parents, parents for their children, the husband for
the help of his wife : ' I am athirst, give me at least one drop
of water. I am still alive. Do not be afraid of me ! ' At
last urged by piety someone placed a mortuary candle at the
head of the sick man and fled from the house." The only
creature that in such distress remained faithful to the end
was the dog. Its devotion is praised in various legends of the
plague.

Centuries later the attitude of the people remained un-
changed, as for instance in the Plague of London in 1665.

When the scourge abated, during a general cleansing of the houses, decomposed corpses were found on all sides, some still in their beds, many beside the beds lying on the floor, they had to be shovelled up ; among them were well-to-do citizens and many opulent merchants. Their servants had forsaken them, their relations had fled, and thus they were overcome by death in the most terrible solitude without food, without attention. A German chronicler states, in regard to the suddenness of death, that many fell down and died without having felt ill before. " On this account many kept a linen cloth in readiness, into which they sewed themselves so soon as they felt the slightest qualm. The corpse-bearers found a woman who had just done this when she was struck down by death. The people fell like flowers at the approach of winter, and the greed for inheritance assumed such proportions that many a one who a short time before had been seen in good health in the street was buried after the elapse of a few hours. A particularly impressive case is reported by Daniel Defoe, the author of *Robinson Crusoe*, who wrote a masterly history of the Plague of London in 1664 and 1665 : " A neighbour and acquaintance of mine, having some money owing to him from a shopkeeper in Whitecross Street, or thereabouts, sent his apprentice, a youth about eighteen years of age, to endeavour to get the money. He came to the door, and, finding it shut, knocked pretty hard, and, as he thought, heard somebody answer within, but was not sure, so he waited, and after some stay knocked again, and then a third time, when he heard somebody coming downstairs.

" At length the man of the house came to the door : he had on his breeches or drawers, and a yellow flannel waistcoat ; no stockings, a pair of slipt shoes, a white cap on his head, and, as the young man said, ' death in his face.'

" When he opened the door, says he : ' What do you disturb me thus for ? ' The boy, though a little surprised, replied : ' I come from such a one, and my master sent me for the money which he says you know of.' ' Very well, child,' returns the living ghost, ' call as you go by at Cripplegate Church, and bid them ring the bell ' ; and with these words he shut the door again, and went up again, and died the same day ; nay, perhaps the same hour."

Reports from different countries and times concerning the suffering caused by the disease vary to an extraordinary extent. Boccaccio makes no reference to pain. Other chroniclers of the fourteenth century report that the sick died within three days gently, as if asleep. Of the children in Germany it is even said that they passed away laughing and singing. In the town of Thornberg the pestilence tormented the people to such a degree that they rent their hands and arms and tore out their hair. In many places in Transylvania they assailed one another in the alleys and streets, and in their frenzy bit and tore each other like dogs and perished miserably.

Defoe relates that the plague-boils, when they grew hard and would not burst, caused such terrible pain that they resembled the most exquisite torture, and that many, to escape their torments, threw themselves out of the windows, shot themselves, or took their own lives in some other way. Very frequently the sufferers became demented from horror and pain. Wrapped in their bed-clothes, they rushed to the graves to bury themselves, as they said. In Provence a man climbed to the roof of his house and hurled the tiles into the street. Another executed a mad grotesque dance on the roof till he was shot down by the guard. A third, who for four days had been lying as if dead, awoke suddenly as a prophet, rushed out into the fields and announced the last judgment, exhorted all to repentance, and cursed those who refused to kneel before him. Such scenes naturally augmented the general horror inspired already by the streets and squares encumbered with corpses. The number everywhere was so great that nowhere were the churchyards sufficient. In Erfurt in 1350 eleven huge trenches were dug and 12,000 corpses were thrown into them. A memorial tablet was placed there. In St. John's churchyard at Nuremberg a gravestone from the year 1437 has been preserved:

> Was that not sad and painful to relate,
> I died with thirteen of my house on the same date?

And from the year 1533:

> Is it not sad and moving to relate,
> I, Hans Tuchmacher, died with fourteen children
> on the same date?

In Swabian Gmuend the inscription on a gravestone in the churchyard of St. Leonard's runs :

> Is that not a painful sight
> Seventy-seven in the same night
> Died of the plague in the year 1637.

To ascertain if anyone was still alive in a house the corpse-bearers in many places threw peas or sand against the windows. If no one appeared they entered the dwelling and fetched out the victims of the plague.

In Italy families of seventy persons were completely exterminated, and many heritages passed over to the fourth heir. In Venice alone no less than fifty Patrician families died out in the year 1348.

The descriptions of the plague from the great cities are particularly heart-rending. " When in London in July 1665 about two thousand died every week, most houses were closed, and the streets were empty. Only great fires were to be seen everywhere, which had been lighted for the purification of the air, and, with the exception of the men who with carts and coffins came to fetch the corpses, no living being was to be seen. On the house doors red crosses were painted with the inscription : ' Lord, have mercy upon us.' Nothing was to be heard save the wailing of the dying, the lamenting of the relations, and the tolling of the bell for those about to be buried, and the mournful call : ' Bring out your dead ! ' "

In Marseilles in 1720 the heaps of corpses were so terrible that the streets became impassable. In front of the door of the heroic bishop Belsunzo there were more than one hundred and fifty corpses, half-decomposed and gnawed by dogs. " The stench proceeding from the corpses quickly decaying in the broiling sun is quite indescribable," Belsunzo writes. " A large number of poor sufferers, in fact whole families, are lying in the open air on straw and wretched mattresses. Some are eagerly awaiting the release of death, some are beside themselves from the consuming heat of the poison. And as if the evil by which they have been attacked were not sufficient, they are further exposed to the most acute suffering by the prevailing famine. One's heart is rent at the sight of so many mothers with the corpses of their children beside

them, whom they must see die off without being able to help
them."

In Vienna also the streets and squares, gardens and vineyards teemed with the sick and dying. " It has been seen,"

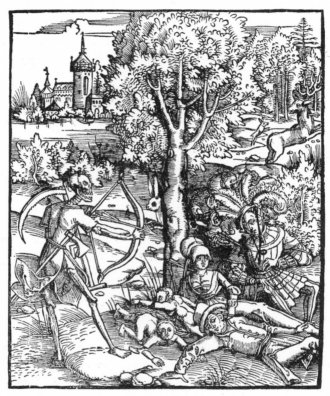

FIGURA MORTIS.
*Anonymous Woodcut from Geiler von Kaisersperg's
" Sermones," 1514.*

writes Abraham a Santa-Clara, " that small children were
found clinging to the breast of the dead mothers where the
innocent little angels could not know that with such drink
they were drinking death. It has been seen that when the
dead mother was placed on the cart her little daughter tried
to accompany her by force, and with a lisping tongue con-

tinued to cry, ' Mammy, mammy,' bringing water to the eyes of the rough, hardened corpse-bearers. It has been seen that in the street near the Imperial Market of Himberg a forsaken little baby boy was found together with a goat, which shaggy nurse the little fellow seemed to be beseeching for a drink in baby manner, in the same way as Romulus and Remus were fostered by a wolf. There have been such a quantity of orphans that they were collected by cart-loads and in the hospital formed a small army of children, most of these were besieging the churchyards where they may easily gain admission, such as had recently lost their mothers and were well on the way of returning to the lap of our common mother, earth." It was terrible to see, whole carts full of nobles and citizens— rich and poor, young and old were led through the streets. When the disease had reached its climax it carried off those infected within twenty-four hours. No one remained to cook, to mind the houses. " Such a one is dead, another dying," was all that was said. The seven gates of the city seem insufficient to allow the dead and sick to pass out. Every day there were intercession services ; every day the bells tolled. To the loud beating of drums high payment was offered to all who would consent to serve as corpse-bearers and sick-attendants. The town-guard had to round up the unemployed of the servant class, lead several surgeons in chains to the hospitals, and ultimately the prisons had to be thrown open and condemned prisoners set to do the repulsive work

No less harrowing than in the cities is the sight offered by the villages and boroughs. In German chronicles we find the same statements as in Boccaccio. Here, too, there is a lack of hands to bury the dead. Here, too, in many places the work of the fields, even the harvest work, had to be suspended, and the cattle strayed from their never-closed byres, abandoned to their own instincts, to return again at night. What the Italian Frari reports from Italy is repeated frequently in the North. " Savage wolves roamed about in packs at night and howled round the walls of the towns. In the villages they did not slake their thirst for human blood by lurking in secret places, as was otherwise their wont, but boldly entered the open houses and tore the little ones from their mothers' sides ;

indeed they did not only attack children, but even armed men and overcame them. To the contemporaries they seemed no longer wild animals but demons. Other quadrupeds forsook their woods, and in herds approached the vicinity of human habitations, as if aware of the extraordinary conditions. Ravens in innumerable flocks flew over the towns with loud croaking. The kite and the vulture were heard in the air, and other unusual migratory birds appeared. But on the houses the cuckoos and owls alighted and filled the night with their mournful lament. The field-mice had lost all fear and took up their abode among human beings."

Descriptions not to be forgotten are those of ships whose whole crews had been carried off by the plague, and which drifted about as derelicts until cast upon some coast where they brought death and destruction to those who hastened to the rescue : that of the simple goose-girl in the East Prussian estate of Przytullen who, as sole survivor of all the inhabitants, delighted in arraying herself in the dresses and jewels of her dead mistress; and thus in the horrible solitude of the forsaken halls of the manor playing the part of the great lady ; that of the young man of Gottersdorf who, hearing that the disease had abated, returned to his village and, on entering, met an old man, who greeted him with the words: "I am the only one of the inhabitants left, and now you come. The plague began at the house of one wicked woman, and at the house of another wicked one at the end of the village it ended." That of the parson in Kerenzen on the Wallenstadt Lake who, when all his congregation were dead, inscribed as last survivor his own name in the register of deaths. Of the inhabitants of the chapter house of Bergen in Norway who had fled to the neighbourhood of Tusededal and there began to build a town, "but the disease pursued them there and carried them all off with the exception of one girl. This girl was discovered some years later, but had run wild and was afraid of human beings, and was therefore called the 'rype,' after a wild bird. But when she had been educated for some time all wildness disappeared. She married, and all the territory in Tusededal which had been marked out for the building of the town was allotted to her and her heirs, who henceforth were known by the name of the 'Rype family.'" Arrid

Hoitfeld relates that many marshes were at this time found
uncultivated which before the time of the " Black Death "
had been ploughed fields, and his book was written three
centuries after the epidemic.

The Black Death and the various outbreaks of plague
have found a staggering, graphic expression in " dance of
death " pictures and engravings and in the numerous " *Icones
Mortis.*" A " dance of death " representation was possessed
practically by every large town. Of those which have been
preserved the most celebrated are those of Luebeck, Basle,
Berne, Strasbourg, Minden, Paris, Dijon, and London.

The experience incorporated in these graphic representations is the equality of all men in the face of death, an
experience of all the greater import as, not only did it shake
the foundations of the rigid system of mediæval castes, but
produced the consciousness of the equality of all men before
the face of God—that consciousness which led up to the
Reformation. If prior to this the higher estimation of the
great had been successfully sustained by the ostentatious
show of their obsequies and the innumerable masses said for
their souls, this deception failed now that even bishops and
prelates frequently remained unburied and their corpses
became the food of dogs, and more essential elements than
external power and position began to assume the first place
in the estimation of men.

To enumerate all the celebrated men carried off by the
plague would take too long. I will only mention a few prominent persons and princes: 1138, Emperor Lothar died of
the plague. 1191, Frederick V, Duke of Swabia. 1270, Louis
the Saint and his son John. 1312, Emperor Henry of Luetzel-
burg. 1349, Emperor Guenther. 1350, the half-brothers of
King Magnus of Sweden, the princes Hakon and Knut, as
well as Alphonso XI, King of Spain. 1352, the Russian
Grand Duke Simeon Ivanovitch the Proud. 1378, Geleazzo
Visconti. 1438, Edward, King of Portugal. 1457, Ladislaus,
King of Bohemia and Hungary. The doges Delfino (1361)
and Michele Morosini (1382). The physicians Guy de Chauliac
(1368), Gentile di Foligno (1348), Cornelio Gemma (1575),
Konrad von Gessner (1565). The painters Pietro and Ambrogio
Lorenzetti (1348), Ghirlandajo (1494), Giorgione (1511),

Perugino (1523), Holbein the Younger (1543), Titian (1576).
The poets Ottavio Salghieri (1630), Friederich Spee (1635),
Opitz von Boberfeld (1639). The founders of Religious Orders,
Bernhard Tolomai (1348) and Gerhard Groote (1384). The
Minister-General of the Franciscan Order, Gerhard Odonis
(1348). The reformer Andreas Bodenstein von Karlstadt (1541).
The originator of Jansenism, Cornelius Jansen (1638). The
great lawyer Johannes Andreae (1348). The philosopher
Hermolas Barbaro (1493). The rhetorician Bruno Cassini
(1348). The historians Giovanni Villani (1348) and Matteo

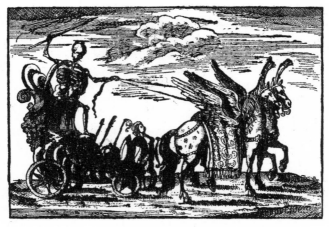

DEATH TRIUMPHANT.
Anonymous Etching of 1711.

Villani (1363). The partisan general Pietro Farnese (1363).
The leader of the Hussites, Johannes Ziska (1421). General
Holk, a character in Schiller's "Wallenstein" (1633). Cardinal
Giovanni Colonna (1348). Archbishop of Spalato, Cucari (1348).
The Archbishops Vassilij of Novgorod and Theognost of Mos-
cow (1352). The Bishop of Paris, Fulques de Chanac (1349);
the Bishop of Luebeck, John IV (1350). The humanist Murrho
(1495).

The number of victims of the plague in the fourteenth
century in Europe is estimated by some to be too low if placed
at 25 per cent. of the population. The number of victims of

later times with vastly superior hygienic and prophylactic conditions must be taken into consideration. Thus in 1467 Moscow mourned the loss of 127,000 victims, Novgorod and district of 230,602, Venice in 1478 of 300,000, Milan 1576, with a population of 200,000 (almost two-thirds of the population are said to have left the town), of 51,000, Berlin in the same year of one-third of its population, Rome of 70,000 in 1591. In Thurgau in 1611 more than half the population died. Milan lost in 1630, 140,000, the Republic of Venice in 1630 and 1631 more than 500,000. In 1630 Cremona was nearly completely depopulated. In Turin there only remained 3,000 persons. In Lorraine, after the plague of 1637, hardly one per cent. of the inhabitants was left. Naples lost in 1635, 300,000. London 160,000 in 1665, Vienna in the year 1579 with a population of 210,000, 123,000, Danzic in 1709 in the course of two months 40,000, Marseilles in 1720, 50,000. Toulon in the same year, with a population of 22,000, 13,160 ; Arles 8,110 from a population of 12,000.

Germany, whose losses for 1348 are estimated at 1,244,434, is one of the countries that suffered least. In Strasbourg there died 16,000 ; in Erfurt, where there were 1,500 deaths on one single day, at least as many. In Basle 14,000, in Weimar 5,000. The losses were particularly great in the North of Germany. In Pomerania (1356) and Holstein two-thirds of the population died, in Schleswig four-fifths. In Luebeck, which at that time was described as the German Venice, it is reported that of 100 inhabitants not 10 survived. The sumtotal is given as 90,000. Hecker is greatly mistaken when he reduces this number to 9,000, as chroniclers report in unison that 1,500 died on a single day. In many German districts only 10 survived out of 100 inhabitants, in quite a number only 5. At Vienna between 500 and 700 died daily. On one day it is reported to have been even 960, and on another 1,200. The chronicler of Salzburg writes : " In Vienna there died daily two or three pounds." Now, a pound comprised 240 pfennig or pence, thus the daily number of deaths was between 480 and 720. In the Certosa of Montrieux of the monks only Gerado, the brother of Petrarch, remained alive. In the monastery of Marienberg in Vinstgau all the monks died with the exception of four. In the same manner nearly all the monks of the monastery of Dissentis were carried off by the plague. At Meiningen the whole convent of the monastery of the Barefooted Friars died out with the exception of three. Altogether there died of the Order of the Franciscans 124,434.

According to Guy de Chauliac three-quarters of the whole population of France died, according to other reports one-half. In many districts, as, for instance, at Viviers and in Burgundy, nine-tenths died. The thoroughly reliable Gilles de Massis relates of towns where out of 20,000 only 200 survived and of smaller towns where out of 1,500 hardly 100. At Avignon two-thirds were carried off. At Montpelier the losses were so immense that it became necessary to grant citizen rights to Italian merchants in order to repopulate the town.

In Italy half the population died. At Venice 100,000, i.e. three-quarters of the population. In order to repopulate the town the doge Orseolo invited foreigners to settle at Venice, offering as enticement the acquirement of citizen rights after two years' residence. Of this invitation it seems many Germans availed themselves. In Genoa six-sevenths died. At Bologna and at Padua two-thirds, at Piacenza one-half, at Pisa seven-tenths. The Prince of Carrarra granted an amnesty to all robbers and criminals who would settle in the deserted towns of Padua and Belluno. Scalinger did the same for Verona, which had lost three-quarters of its population. At Siena there died 80,000. At Florence, with a population of roughly 130,000 inhabitants, according to Boccaccio more than 100,000 died. According to Petrarch's report hardly 10 out of 100 survived. From London it was reported that scarcely every tenth man survived. The number of deaths is said to be underestimated at 100,000. At Bristol hardly one-tenth of the population remained. At Norwich out of a population of 70,000 there died 57,374. In England of the clergy alone there died 25,000. From the town of Smolensk in Russia in 1386 there remained only five persons alive. The islands of Cyprus and Iceland are said to have been depopulated to the last inhabitant.

APPENDICES

A Letter from Naples of July 10, 1656

"The town is now only recognisable by its edifices and magnificent houses and no longer by its teeming population, the decrease and destruction of which is constantly augmented by the piled-up corpses, of which 60,000 were burned—one part on Sunday morning and one part on Wednesday night. 170,000 have further been buried in huge trenches, the most aristrocratic in the churches. The air is always so thick and misty, and is further obscured by multitudes of birds enticed by the carrion of the corpses, the stench of which is overwhelming. The dead are no longer counted. Misery and grief are great and general. Nearly all who are infected die, no one escapes. And those who survive the plague are killed by the famine. To avoid this latter many a nobleman is seen going about without a cloak with a bundle of wood on his back, bearing home bread, vegetables, wine, and other provisions, as there is a shortage of servants, all of whom are dead; and it is necessary to procure food with the sweat of one's brow and weigh it with diamond scales, although it is of a nature that even the sight of it causes horror, to say nothing of eating it.

"The most beautiful girls have now abandoned all pretensions to magnificent clothes, but are seen scurrying through the streets like shadows in search of food they are unable to find. Could they but only procure a little oil that they can have a light at night, so as not to have to die in the dark, like so many in the houses without the assistance of friends or servants, who die of starvation or are carried off by the plague and thus buried alive in their own houses. Gold and silver and costly furniture no longer possess the power to purchase bread.

"In the house next to ours a nobleman died last Sunday who had lost all his servants by the disease. His wife and a cousin were still alive, but in the course of two days they died too, as they had nothing to eat or drink—they simply fell back on their beds and were found dead in their own beds.

"In our neighbourhood there used to live more than a thousand nobles and rich people, of whom but five remain— a woman, three children, and a priest—but all are infected, and our house stands in the midst of them. In spite of this, by the grace of God, we are all still healthy, and as if by a miracle of God and by His grace are still alive.

"In consequence of the scourge more than 10,000 people in this town are said to be dead, and, in spite of this, many continue to die, and it seems as if the Almighty had decreed our complete destruction.

"I have written a great deal, but have hardly succeeded in giving an idea of the misery. All kinds of people are to be seen here, who have lost their senses, running about in their shirts or even completely naked. In their distress they often fall down in the streets and die.

"All that is heard is woeful weeping, fit to cause the deepest pity. The people are perishing, and there is such an abominable stench that it alone would suffice to kill, so that everyone longs for death, to be delivered from this fearful misery. Many die in despair, believing that hell can be no worse. Multitudes of dogs and cats scamper through the streets, appeasing their hunger on the corpses lying about everywhere. The churches, shops, and houses are all closed. There are neither doctors, physicians, apothecaries, nor priests to be had; thus all must die without medical attention or sacrament. Those who are fortunate are dragged with a rope round their necks to a field and burnt. The others remain lying in the streets and alleys, and are gnawed by dogs and cats. Thus we are suffering greater persecution and humiliation than the Jews under Titus Vespasianus, because we have deserved it more than they by our great sins. May God preserve the master in His mercy, and I submit my soul to the Almighty God.

"Thy devoted
JOHN BAPTISTA SPINELL.

"Post Scriptum. Dated Rome, October 17th:

"The plague here is daily on the increase and nearly three hundred people die every day. In Naples the Viceroy is preparing a list describing all houses left ownerless, so as to acquire for the King the fortunes of those who have no blood relations. More than three hundred thousand people have died there, of whom sixty thousand have been burnt and twenty thousand have been thrown into the sea, as there was no one left to bury them."

COPY OF A DOLEFUL LETTER FROM DANZIC OF THE 22ND OF OCTOBER, 1709

" I cannot refrain from conveying to you with sorrow-laden pen a woeful account of our miserable condition which to our great misfortune has overwhelmed us with great intensity. The hand of God has for nearly two months lain heavily on us by the fearful plague, and has chastised us so heavily that already, according to the local lists supplied weekly by the gravediggers, more than forty thousand people have passed away. Day and night the mournful bell is heard tolling, and in every street one is met by coffins, some borne by hand, others upon carts or simply dragged along, which is a pitiful sight to see. Not far from my lodgings a stout woman who had died was being carried away, and, perhaps, because the bearers were too weak, they stumbled with the coffin, which flew from their shoulders and broke to pieces, so that the naked corpse fell out, revealing such a fearful sight that it so frightened one of the bearers that he immediately sank dead to the ground.

" In all the streets nothing is heard but weeping and wailing, and one is half-choked by the horrible smoke of the plague powder, which is frequently burnt in many places. The doors and lower windows of most of the houses are nailed up, and those who live in them have handed up to them what they require to sustain their life, and those who require anything let down baskets by ropes from the upper windows and draw up what has been placed in them. Of the whole Town Council here only two are still alive, the others are all dead. And only nine of our clergy are still alive, five of our vergers and four of our medical men. The principal Patricians have gone; the best-known houses, both noble and *bourgeois*, have been devastated by the plague, and there are only fifty-eight houses in which the gruesome scourge has not raged. My lodgings are among these. My pen is incapable of describing how wretched things are here everywhere. There are people here who do not leave the church the whole day, but put a little bread and a bottle of beer into their pockets and from morning till evening remain at prayers, till they return to go to bed, and this they do day after day. In the churches only people in deep mourning are seen, no coloured dress or bright ribbon. The whole time the people are on their knees, weeping, praying, and whining so miserably that it would melt a stone. No one is sure of his life for a single hour, for he may die at his meals, at his work, at home, at church, or in the street. In short, everywhere they are exposed to the arrow of death. In our house, thank God, all have remained well and healthy, except our maid, who, being sent to purchase bread, did not return, so that we do not know if she is dead or has met with some other misfortune. The manner in which people are affected is not always the same. For many people die a terrible death in the worst excesses of raving madness; they rush about the streets in their shirts and rave so terribly that one's hair stands on end.

" Although one might think that the proximity of death would act as a deterrent from sin, yet desperate minds seem to be encouraged by the scourge of death to still greater misdeeds. For great wickedness is committed by godless men who turn to robbing and stealing and secretly slip into the houses. In cases where they know that there is something worth stealing and only one or two persons alive in the house, they ill-treat them or even murder them, and take possession of what they desire. The houses are searched daily, morning and evening; the dead are carried out and the sick handed over to the care of the plague doctors. It frequently happens that in a single day and night more than a hundred people are buried, of whom a few are provided with coffins; but the majority are simply placed in a grave 12, 20, 30, even 50 together, piled up above one another—and I have often heard that the people are frequently not quite dead and are yet carried away by the impatient gravediggers like so many carcases. Alas! my pen revolts with grief and horror, for our daily life is fearful, and we would fain desire that places and

towns as yet untouched by God's avenging hand should see
and know one tenth part of our misery or could cast but one
glance at our unhappy town, they would certainly be amazed
and dumbfoundered with terror, and day and night, pray to
God graciously to preserve them from the plague.

"In short, I am in God's hands and do not know if I shall
live till to-morrow, and therefore I am constantly prepared
that I may be ready to do God's will, and, as I am by no means
sure that this will not be the last letter I may be able to write,

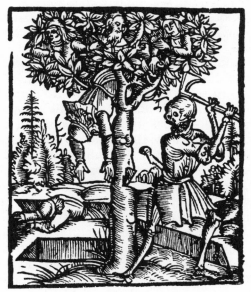

DEATH FELLING THE TREE OF LIFE.
*Anonymous Woodcut from Geiler von Kaisersperg's
"Sermones," 1514.*

I take leave of you in this world, wishing you all prosperity
both in this world and in the life to come."

CIRCUMSTANTIAL NARRATIVE OF THE PLAGUE AT VIENNA
AND OF THE DISTRESSFUL TIME
(*Abraham a Santa-Clara*)

The "Black Death" originated in the Leopold Town
quarter, which a few years ago, on account of its wicked

population, was known as the Jewish Town, and had there for some time been consuming the population, but in a moderate degree ; subsequently the plague stole across the Danube, or rather over an arm of the Danube, to the other suburbs, and at first it appeared as if the scourge did not venture to penetrate into the residence, but would rest content with raging in the suburbs, as it had already devastated them thoroughly ; however, in such a manner that it was mostly the dirty localities which were assailed by this evil, and only the lower orders, as well as the rabble, of which no town is void, who fell victims to the scythe of death ; so that it was not untruthfully said that death was only carrying off the chaff, searching the beggars' sacks, was going to appease his appetite with common bread, and that the aristocratic houses and dwellings of the rich would probably be safeguarded against his scythe. " Ha, ha," quoth Death, " that ye may know that no fortress can resist me and even if it had bastions like the Ditzberg in Carinthia, the Schoeckl in Styria, the Chasteiner in Salzburg, the Caravancas in Bavaria, the Leberberg in Switzerland, the Fichtelberg in Bohemia, the Kallenberg in Austria, etc., and if it were surrounded by a moat which could supply water to the mighty ocean, in spite of all this I will take the town." And this, unfortunately, he did in July, and in August carried out the general plundering and gruesome sacking !

In the times of Cæsar the Dictator an ox opened its mouth and spoke in Rome. In the time of the Prophet Balaam a she-ass spoke. In the time of the Emperor Mauritius a metal statue spoke. In the time of Tarquinius Superbus a dog spoke. In the time of the venerable Bede a stone spoke. But at this time at Vienna, as at this corner, a sick man was lying, on the other side a dying man was groaning, a few steps further a dead man was stretched, and the corpses on the public streets barred the way of the cart-drivers, the streets spoke after this fashion, exhorting all to repentance and penance : " Arise, arise, O ye sinful ! The axe has already been laid to the tree, the wrath of God is at the gate, the voice of the Most High is summoning you to Eternity, the archangel Michael already holds the scales in which your works are to be weighed. Arise, arise, and in the few fleeting hours which still remain do penance ; for this alone is the

sponge which can wipe out your sins, this alone is the fire
which can consume your sinful account, this alone is the branch
which can preserve you from falling into eternal damnation.
Tears of repentance, believe, are the only *aqua fortis* which
can destroy the chains by which you are bound to the service
of the wicked fiend.   The throbs of a penitent heart, in that
you may trust, may yet burst open the gates of heaven closed
against you.   The contrite sighs, in that you may place
confidence, are the only music which can appease the wrath
of God.   Arise, arise, make ready for your journey to Eternity,
so that, although you must surrender your temporal life, you
may not at least, at the same time, lose your eternal life.
Arise, arise, ye all, also, innocent men, for thus is the decree
of the Most High that, although by a Christian course of life
ye have not called down the wrath of God, all the same many
of you must accompany the wicked to Eternity.   Purge your-
selves, therefore, of the slight blemishes, without which we
miserable children of Adam are unable to exist, so that you
may escape temporal punishment."   It was in this fashion
that the streets and roads spake unto us, and the plaster on
which we trod with our feet reminded all that they forthwith
should seek a plaster for the wounds of their conscience, as
with amazement it was seen that the people hastened to the
churches and with streaming eyes fell at the feet of the confessors, thus preparing themselves for death ; and many hundreds of these had hardly left the churches and the altars and
were on the way to their homes when the hand of God touched
them, causing boils and spots upon their bodies—yea that even
many of them fell suddenly to the ground before the confes-
sionals, so that, half dead, they had to be dragged out of the
doors ; and some few, who still preserved a spark of courage,
assembled in the public streets, but with their nostrils wrapped
in fumigated kerchiefs—no longer announcing, as in former
times, what news the courier had brought from the empire, nor
tidings from Madrid, but only the mournful report of present
misery; and when after hasty discourse they took leave of one
another their eyes filled with tears, as if foreboding told them
that on the third day they would not see each other more.

The inns are usually a resort of merriment, occasionally
too of excesses ; for it is well known that when the Blessed

Virgin arrived at Bethlehem with Joseph they had to seek shelter in a draughty stable, there being no room for them in the inn ; and it is true that in such houses our most benevolent Lord at the present time can find no room, because all is overcrowded with wickedness.   That a swine should be born of a lamb, a raven of an eagle, a goat of a horse is not so pro-digious a marvel ; for experience has rendered such happenings familiar to us.   Who has not heard that men by drink at the " White Lamb " have been converted into swine, at the " Golden Eagle " into gallow birds, at the " Red Horse " into licentious goats ; let not this astonish you, for when Bacchus plies the bellows Venus sits by the fireside.   But this does not apply to all inns, but only to such which in their accommoda-tion include both wine and women.   Inns, in short, are in many cases brothels, and in no other place does the piper reap a richer harvest for his inciting tune, and all montebanks and clowns can here dispose of their wares in return for gleaming silver—but at that time in populous Vienna the sad reverse of merriment was seen, and many a potman had more to do in making up a reckoning not of what had been drunk, but of the drinkers whom in the morning he found either before or behind the door—yea, frequently host and guests were borne away together on the corpse cart.   The floor which formerly had to be sprayed to lay the dust for dancing was now sprayed with tears; nor did the hosts need to rinse the glasses with cool water to keep them whole, but their thoughts were more occupied with preserving their lives, which were more fragile than their glass; instead of sweet draughts they drew deep sighs, and there was more to be seen—oh transformation—of whining than of wine !

And people walked the streets as if deprived of heart and stricken dumb, and their pale faces bore witness of the state of their internal works.   Occasionally in some street the greeting was heard: "Well met, dear brother, are you still alive ? " and to this came the answer with the addition said in a half-broken voice : " Yes, yes, I am still alive, but my father, my mother, my sister, all are dead," which deprived conversation of all further voice, and tear-filled eyes alone bade still farewell.

In the year 1578 the town of Lisbon was in great distress,

nearly seventy thousand people had died ! Hard set was the
town of Breslau in Silesia in 1542, where in the course of
twenty-two weeks five thousand nine hundred people had been
carried off. A sorry sight was then offered by Rome, where
on a single day ten thousand people died. Indescribable
tribulation descended on Prague in 1381, so that on a single
day there died one thousand one hundred and sixteen men,
as Hedius reports. In 1466 the town of Paris suffered a great
scourge of dying, during which in a short time nearly forty
thousand citizens were laid in the earth. Terrible misery
overcame the town of Venice in 1576, when within nine months
nearly sixty thousand people were carried off by death. Thus
it may be seen that these towns were assailed with great
misfortune ; but he who lived in the year 1679, in the Wien
quarter of Vienna in the month of September, he must proclaim
that to depict such misery surpasses the art of all painters,
for the ravages of death were such that many thought the
general epilogue and end of the whole world had come—there
is not a single street or by-lane, of which there are so many
in this populous capital, in which death did not rage. In
Lord Street death was overlord. In Prudence Street he was
not prudent but lavish. In Bow Street he shot down all.
In Singer Street he sang a requiem for many. No holiday
did he grant in School Street. In Strap Street he cut straps
out of the skins of many. No saint's day was there in Saint
Dorothea Street. In Lieber, Briener, Kaerner, Donfalt,
Wiplinger Highways death was the highway robber ; in Nailor
Street death put new points upon his arrows ; in Heaven Gate
Street death sent many a one to heaven or, perhaps, somewhere else. In the High Market death laid many low. In
the Fish Market death observed no fasts. In the New Market
death did nothing new. In Coal Market death caused all to
don coal-black weeds. In the Tinder Market death set all
ablaze. In the Peasants' Market death found many citizens.
In the Butchers' Market death had his meat stall. In the
Sow Market, now called Show Market, death made a good
display. In the Moat death's works were not remote. In
the Space death worked apace. In the Heathens' Range death
shot down many Christians. In the Jews' Square death did
a good deal. In Ropers' Walk death laid snares for many.

In the Fire Scene death burnt many so that they turned to dust and ashes. In Salt Gate death oversalted many a life ! In the Cat Climb death caught many a mouse. The Pig Corner death cleared out thoroughly. In the Twelve Apostles death played Iscariot. In the Green Meadow death dried up many like the grass to hay, *omnis caro fœnum.* St. Peter's Graveyard death left as a graveyard. From the High Bridge death hurled down many a one. In the " Fire Side " the cold sweat of death passed over many a brow. In " Locksmith Lane " death opened many a door leading to Eternity. In "Maiden Lane " death played the gallant. In " Bushel Lane " death did not put his light under a bushel, but raged openly in the face of all. " Wheel Lane " was no wheel of luck against death. In " Rose Lane " death broke many roses. In " Jews' Lane " death kept no Sabbath. In " Blood Lane " death did not blush crimson red. In " Race Lane " few outpaced death. In " Straw Lane " he strangled many on their straw bedding. In " Dyers' Lane " death dyed most with the pale hue of death. In " Inn Lane " death's cup did not spare many. On " Crown Hill " death wielded his sceptre. At " Fishermen's Steps " many were caught in death's net. In " Willow Borough " death behaved like a sheriff. In " Stick and Trap " death proved inexorable.

In short, there is no street nor road, although their names are not all mentioned here, both in Vienna and in its great, broad spreading suburbs, which was not devastated by the rage of death. For the whole month in Vienna and around it nothing else was to be seen but corpses being borne away, driven away, dragged away to burial; yea and the distress grew so great that, as many hands were required, the hard-set town had for many weeks to recruit gravediggers to the public beat of drums, and mournful was the sound of these drums and to many caused a painful pang, so that hardly one was to be found in a thousand for this gruesome task, for which a surfeit of wages was offered; on which account all prisons, jails, and penitentiaries in which many were detained were carefully searched, and those who had by crime forfeited their lives according to judicial sentence were pressed to do this work, and most of them, escaping from the iron bonds of prison, fell under the scythe of death.

CHAPTER II

THE PRECURSORS OF THE PLAGUE

Hippocrates—Relapse to paganism—Luther's superstition—Mischief of spectres and rogues—Astrology—Prophecies in Russia—Fateful comets—Mastersinger Hans Folz—Snakes, locusts, and other vermin—Abortions—Spectral funerals—Small crosses and drops of blood rain from the sky—A forefather of modern journalism—Prophets and predictions of the end of the world.

Appendix : " Did death dispatch certain precursors to Vienna to announce his arrival ? " (Abraham a Santa-Clara).

ALREADY Hippocrates maintained that in the plague there was something of a divine origin, transcending human conception.

As up to the beginning of the seventeenth century this opinion was held by the medical authorities, it may easily be conceived with what terror the people were inspired by the divine scourge which in various places was actually described as " God's disease." In all places where popular imagination was not diverted into ecclesiastic channels the demons of heathen times, which still persisted in tradition, again gained mastery over the popular mind.

In Bavaria the people at the time of the " Black Death " made nocturnal pilgrimages with torches and candles to the Peninsula of the " Three Ladies " in the Kochel Lake, and there worshipped in the subterranean passages " The Three " : Einbett (One Bed) Wollbett (Woollen Bed) and Vilbett (Many Beds). At that time, also, the stone statues of Saint Einbede, Saint Warbede, and Saint Villebede were erected in the cathedral of Worms.

In Rome, in the plague year 1522, a Greek, Demetrius, walked through the town with a bull which had been tamed by witchcraft, and sacrificed it according to ancient custom before the eyes of all the people at the Colosseum to propitiate the hostile demons. In Lower Lusatia, in the year 1612, the following custom prevailed among the Wend peasantry : Nine persons were selected—two young chaste farm labourers, a widow who had lived seven years in widowhood, and six pure maidens. These forgathered at midnight at the end of the village. One labourer brought a plough on four oxen; another a rod of dead wood—with this he described a circle, into which the seven women stepped and in which they divested themselves of all their clothing. Then the widow proceeded carrying the rod, the maidens harnessed themselves to the plough and drew a furrow round the whole village, followed by one of the labourers, the other remaining to guard the clothes. When the work was completed they returned home without uttering a word. This custom of ploughing round the village, by which it was believed that a barrier was set up against evil powers, persisted in the central and southern Volga Government and in Siberia in 1890.

The belief in devils and spirits was also greatly stimulated by the plague. Even such a man as Martin Luther shared the opinion that all pestilence was brought upon the people by evil spirits, " that they poisoned the air or otherwise infected the poor people by their breath and injected the mortal poison into their bodies." Thus in nearly all countries we meet with the belief in the " plague virgin," who only needs to raise her hand to scatter the plague poison. The spirit was seen in the shape of a blue flame flying through the air and developing on the lips of the dying and dead. Those who saw it rushed away calling " Run, the owlet is coming." As recently as the beginning of last century the Lithuanian peasants are said to have sung a ballad to the following effect : " In a small town the ' plague virgin ' once appeared, in accordance with her custom she stroked the doors and windows with her hand and made her red scarf flutter in the wind. The inhabitants shut themselves up carefully in their houses, but hunger and other necessities obliged them to go out from time to time and thus expose themselves to death. Then a young nobleman, although sufficiently provided with stores and able to sustain a long siege by the ' plague virgin,' resolved to sacrifice himself for the salvation of his fellow citizens. He took his broadsword, which was inscribed with the motto

' Jesus and Mary,' and boldly opened the door. When the hand of the spirit appeared he cut it off and took possession of the red scarf." The result may be guessed. The nobleman died as well as his family. But since then the little town has never again had to suffer from any visitation of the plague. As late as the seventeenth and beginning of the eighteenth centuries it was endeavoured to exclude the white spirit of the plague from the houses by spinning threads across the openings of doors and windows. A Finnish song conjures the plague to depart with all haste to the steel-hard mountains, to the dark North—horses and carriage are to be provided for the journey. In effigy the plague was burnt, buried, immured, banished in temples and churches. And it appeared not only as a wandering or blind woman, but rode as a man on a black horse, sailed as a black man on ships and barks ; it was a bad walker and contrived to be driven into the villages or carried on someone's back ; with a broom it swept in front of the houses, and where it had swept all people died.

But a great variety of superstitions are connected with the plague ; thus it is reported from the year 1654 " that two spirits, a good one and a bad one, were seen walking about. The latter, the bad one, carried, like a huntsman, a boar spear in his hand ; the former, the good spirit, a sword ; when the good spirit pointed out a house to him, he beat against it with his spear, and as many blows as he struck so many people died in the house on the following day." In the year 1682 it is said that death was seen and heard in human form at Spandau, " where he climbed over the garden gate of some old women, settled on a bench as if asleep, but soon woke up again, thanked for the hospitality, gave his name, and said that he was death and they should not be alarmed if he should create a stir in the neighbourhood. In Stendal he walked about and talked, and patted a girl engaged to be married on her head and promised her security."

" In Brandenburg there appeared in 1559 horrible men, of whom at first fifteen and later on twelve were seen. The foremost had beside their posteriors little heads, the others fearful faces and long scythes, with which they cut at the oats, so that the swish could be heard at a great distance, but the oats remained standing. When a quantity of people came running out to see them, they went on with their mowing. This was interpreted by the scholars, on an enquiry of the Elector, as an indication of a speedy outbreak of an epidemic, which then took place and in which the tall mower death cut down many men."

That such apparitions were not always only the results of optical illusions, but that mentally and morally deranged men frequently endeavoured to terrify the public by all kinds of trickery, is borne out by a series of legal prosecutions. Thus a woman was pilloried at Thorn and punished with fifteen strokes of the rod, because during an epidemic of plague she wandered about the suburbs dressed in white declaring she was death. In consequence of the frequency with which the outbreaks succeeded one another from the fourteenth to the seventeenth centuries—an outbreak may be recorded nearly every twenty years, frequently every ten years—the minds of the people were highly excited and strained. Numerous other epidemics, earthquakes, famines, wars, and plagues of vermin contributed still further, so that they were daily in expectation of terrible events. A great rôle was played by the indications and precursors which, according to popular belief, preceded such happenings. Above all, it was the constellations which determined the destiny of man, and particular positions of the planets were regarded as the direct cause of the plague. For this, support was found in the principle authority of the mediæval ages—in Aristotle, who regarded the conjunction of Mars and Jupiter as specially menacing. Thus the outbreak of the great plague in 1348 was preceded by the conjunction of Saturn, Jupiter, and Mars under the fourteenth degree of Aquarius, on March 20, 1345, at 1 p.m. Later on this conjunction has always been regarded as the true cause of the plague : " For one (Saturn) collects the evil vapours in the depth of the earth, the other draws them up into the heights of the air, particularly when the moon is subject to eclipse in the sign of Aquarius, the Scales, or the Scorpion. Such an eclipse took place on April 15, 1679. On this day there was the first case of plague in the Leopold's Town quarter of Vienna." That Saturn in Aquarius was regarded as giving rise to plague was stated in the foundation document of the University of Wittenberg, and many were of opinion that

Saturn was the horseman on the pale horse. In the year 1447 the celebrated physician, Marsilius Ficinus, then aged a hundred and eight years, prophesied from the conjunction of the planets Saturn and Jupiter together with other signs

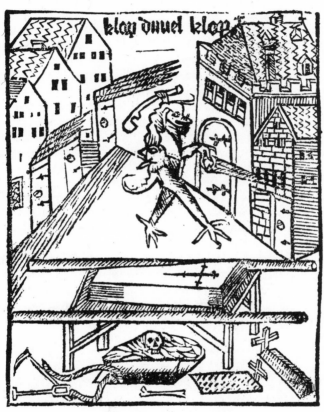

"KNOCK, DEVIL, KNOCK."
Printed at Cologne, 1508.

and constellations the plague which arrived two years later, " carrying off even cats and dogs." In the year 1664 the astrologer, Dr. Engelhardt, predicted to Czar Alexei Michailo-vitch for the year 1665 a terrible plague which would affect more countries than Russia. This bold prophecy was actually fulfilled, and the terrible outbreak in London in 1665 caused

terror and horror in all countries, and particularly there where
this pretended prophecy had drawn attention to the fearful
event. Intercourse was, therefore, prohibited with foreign
countries at all frontiers by an express order of the Czar. The
port of Archangel was closed, and even such foreigners who
arrived at Plesskov and Novgorod from the Swedish frontier
were subjected to a severe examination and were not allowed
to proceed to Moscow without special permission of the Czar.

As particular instigators and precursors of all great universal plagues the comets were regarded, which in the centuries
when these epidemics were most prevalent were extraordinarily frequent. In the period from 1298 to 1314 seven were
enumerated, twenty-six between 1500 and 1543, fifteen or sixteen between 1556 and 1597. Frequently several appeared one
after another every year. For the year 1618 alone the number
is stated to have been eight or nine. Seneca had already
declared comets to be malicious apparitions, preceding
disease, civil strife, war, and earthquake. Hippocrates and
Avicenna, the two chief medical authorities, taught that:
"Comets, auroras, and particularly eclipses of the sun and
moon, were the cause and precursors of future pestilences."
Aristotle had explained the comets as apparitions of the air
due to exhalations of the earth, and the Mastersinger of
Nuremberg, Hans Folz, in his rhymes of the plague of 1482,
attributes their baneful effect to their power of extracting all
moisture :

> . . . and comets with their fiery tails,
> In Germany as dry stars they are known,
> And everywhere that one has flown
> From that same land all moisture it withdraws,
> Which from all things it takes by Nature's laws,
> From men, from beasts, from earth,
> So that they are deprived, and dearth
> Must suffer of their vital essence
> Which causes drought, fever, and excrescence.
> This may be seen, as is revealed quite clear
> By war, great plague, or famine year—
> This too is cause of the foul atmosphere.

Comets were also said to be God's letters of renunciation or
his chastisement rods. " In 1117, in January, a comet passed

like a fiery army from the North towards the Orient, the moon was o'ercast blood-red in an eclipse, a year later a light appeared more brilliant than the sun.   This was followed by great cold, famine, and plague, of which one-third of humanity is said to have perished.   At this time a child lying swaddled in its cradle at Cremona is said to have addressed its mother by her name, and to have related that it had seen the Holy Virgin Mary beseeching her son that he would not destroy the world ;

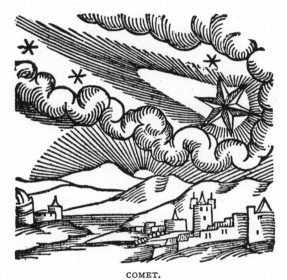

COMET.

From the Chronicle of Marvels of Conradus Lycosthenes.

hereafter the child spake never a word till the rightful time had come."

A particularly terrible comet, of awe-inspiring blackness, is said to have preceded the outbreak of the " Black Death " in Europe.   Again, in the year 1618, a large comet spread general terror, and was regarded as the precursor of the calamity which overtook the world fourteen years later.   Pope Urban VIII found it necessary to institute public prayers and a jubilee for the purpose of allaying the public anxiety.   " What wretchedness and misery," an author writes in 1683, " has been brought about in this century alone, in which we live, by comets?   And now we have the plague-announcer, the comet, before our very eyes. It stands above our heads, *Flagellium Dei*, the Scourge of God, Attila, a cruel tyrant and king of the Huns was called. Oh, who can tell what punishment this comet which God has sent may mean ? " Here again the relation of the comet to the other constellations was of particular significance. From this could be determined what country, what people, what animals had most to fear from the comet and the nature of the evil threatened. A comet in the Ram signified grievous wars, deadly epidemics, the fall of the mighty and the rise of the lowly ; great drought in places situated in the realm of this tropic. In the Virgin it signified premature and dangerous delivery of pregnant women, heavy taxation, imprisonment, and death of many women. In the Scorpion it meant, in addition to the above evils, insect plagues and locusts in innumerable hosts. In the Fishes, religious strife, terrible disturbances of the atmosphere, war, plague, and most certainly death of the mighty. The dread of comets was so deeply rooted in human imagination that no one dared to advance arguments to pacify the anxiety of the people at the comet of 1618. The celebrated mathematician, Jacques Bernoulli, got out of the difficulty in a discussion with upholders of the mission of comets by declaring: "The crown of the comet could not be a sign of divine anger, because it was of eternal nature, but the tail of the comet might well admit of this interpretation." Thus Peter Bayle's treatise—"Various considerations on the occasion of the Comet of 1680"—was an act of great scientific and moral courage and a literary sensation of the first order. When Halley had established the nature of comets as stars and had predicted the reappearance of the particularly brilliant comet of 1682 for the year 1758, and his calculation had proved to be right, the constellations of planets and the appearance of comets had to be suppressed in the predictions of plagues.

In addition to comets there were all kinds of other fiery signs which were considered as precursors of the plague. Thus on December 20, 1348, there stood at dawn a column of fire above the palace of the Pope at Avignon, and in August of the same year there was seen above Paris a ball of fire which remained visible for a considerable time. To this category belongs an event which happened in Austria, at Vienna, in the year 1568, "When in sun and moonlight a beautiful rainbow and a fiery beam were seen hovering above the church of St. Stephanie, which was followed by a violent epidemic in Austria, Swabia, Augsburg, Wuertemberg, Nuremberg, and other places, carrying off human beings and cattle." Further stinking mists, rains of snakes and frogs, storms and floods, earthquakes, famines and locusts, were all considered as precursors of the plague. Hecker, in his celebrated book on

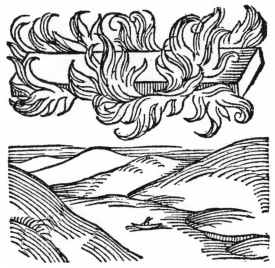

FIERY BEAM FALLS FROM THE SKY.
From Lycosthenes.

the "Black Plague," 1832, and Haeser, in his "Historical Pathological Enquiries," 1839, by no means question the causal connection of the cosmic and telluric events with the outbreak of the plague. "The most terrific revolutions in the existence of the earth, floods, volcanic eruptions, tempests, heavy, moist pestilential fogs (a feature which preceded the epidemic nearly throughout its whole course)—these products of an outburst of the inorganic forces of Nature, to which in the lower organic life of Nature as a parallel feature the production of innumerable swarms of insects (Chinese reports even mention

a rain of snakes), the failure of crops, etc., may be added—
served as an introduction to the plague, so far as its extent is
known, particularly in the place of its first origin, China."

Particularly violent earthquakes preceded the "Black
Death" of 1348 in 1347. At Venice the earthquake was so
violent that the bells of St. Mark began to ring and whole
towers and churches collapsed.

As the plague was in the first instance attributed to the
vitiation of the air, the plague-engendering nature of the

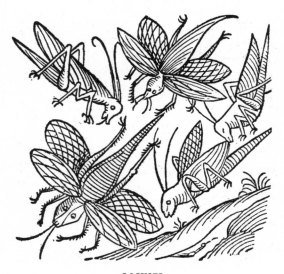

LOCUSTS.
From Lycosthenes.

locusts was evident. The horribly stinking vermin used to lie
a foot high in the ponds and wells, and their filth dripped as
an oily, stinking mass from the roofs. The famine which in
consequence of the lack of means of communication and the
prejudice existing against commerce in corn invariably
followed every inroad of locusts also tended to weaken the
constitutions and to render them more susceptible to an
epidemic of plague. Already St. Augustine relates of a fearful
plague which was announced by swarms of locusts. Towards
the end of June 1338 there appeared coming from Asia swarms

of migratory locusts in such numbers that they darkened the sun and, if they alighted, covered the ground for several miles round. With the exception of the vines everything in the fields was devoured. Only three years later were they completely eradicated. Again, in the year 1346 the locusts and white mice had announced the plague in Germany. " In 1478 the whole of Latin Europe was plagued by locusts which devastated everything, gardens, meadows and fields, after which a great epidemic came into the land, and in Venice alone there died more than 300,000 persons."

" Memorable for the year 1335 is the pernicious inroad of locusts which, coming through Poland, Bohemia, and Austria from the East, penetrated into the Empire. As described by Aventinus, these soldiers possessed six wings each and teeth which gleamed like precious stones. They flew so thick in the air that they darkened the sun and cast a shadow on the earth. They always dispatched a vanguard a day before which, so to say, had to find quarters for the main body and select a place for their encampment—a word very applicable to this invasion, as it was indeed a war against the fields, whose leaves and grass, flowers and seed, stalks and herbs were bitten off and consumed by these hosts ; but, as Bonfinius relates, the vineyards were spared. They were seemingly divided into regiments—they rose at dawn and did not descend to the ground till nine o'clock. Monsignor Carl in Moravia once endeavoured to measure the extent of their camp and found that its breadth amounted to 35,000 paces or three German miles, but it was impossible to ride along its full length in a single day. In winter they crept into holes to reappear next summer ; this was carried on for four successive summers. In Bavaria someone raised an army of fowls to encounter them, but the more they destroyed and swallowed of these uninvited guests the more there came up to take their places. At last the storks, ravens, vultures, and magpies fell upon them in the fourth year and destroyed the majority ; the rest were smothered by a thick snow which fell upon them."

Just as the rotting locusts were held responsible for the plague, so were all other extensive sources of putrefaction by which the air was infected. Thus Forestus Alcmarianos relates that he himself saw a whale " 28 ells in length and

14 ells broad which, coming from the western sea, was thrown
upon the shore of Egemont by great waves and was unable to
reach the open again ; it produced so great a foulness and
malignity of the air that very soon a great epidemic broke out
in Egemont and neighbourhood."

Further indications are unusual insects, strange worms,
big-bellied toads, unknown frogs with tails with which the
medical men of the period were not familiar, large quantities
of all kinds of beetles, large, black vineyard moths, large
spiders, gnats " of uncanny shape and colour." " Further,
when snakes, bats, badgers, and other animals, which dwell in
deep holes in the earth, come out in the fields in great multitudes and forsake their ordinary dwellings ; when the fruit and
leguminous plants become very rotten and full of worms, when
poisonous fungi sprout up, when the fields and woods are full
of spider webs ; when cattle fall ill or even die on the pastures,
as well as the wild animals in the woods, when bread readily
turns mouldy and mildewed. Newly developed flies, worms,
and midges are observed on the snow, the fruit and other crops
fail to mature or rot, disease is observed particularly in sheep
and swine, dogs go mad, many move about like shadows on
the wall, black vapours are observed to rise from the earth
like a mist, the ravens are prompted by unusual impulses and
fly round the hospitals in pairs. In the neighbourhood of
water there is for a full hour a sound of washing and beating of
clothes at night which is heard quite close, and it has been
observed that this is indicative of an epidemic among women.
Birds, contrary to their habits, are restless at night, fly about
hither and thither, certain birds called plague birds appear,
some maintain that a ghost with a voice like some lowing
domestic animal is heard, frogs sit huddled together in
scores or one on the top of the other, in the hospitals and sick
houses a great rushing wind is heard, and when one perceives
among men a great lack of reliability, jealousy, and hatred and
wantonness, if then the plague does not ensue, some other
inscrutable disease that is difficult to cure is sure to come. If
newly baked bread is placed for the night at the end of a pole
and in the morning is found to be mildewed and internally
grown green, yellow and uneatable, and when thrown to fowls
and dogs causes them to die from eating it, in a similar manner

if fowls drink the morning dew and die in consequence, then the plague poison is near at hand. Nor are extraordinary things both visible and invisible at all times to be considered diabolical machinations, superstition or idolatry, but may be regarded as the work of God."

Further precursory indications are when pregnant women frequently produce abortions, when plaintive wailing is heard in graveyards, when funerals are seen passing in the clouds, when children in their playgrounds play at funeral processions. " During the whole of the year 1382 there was no wind, in consequence of which the air grew putrid, so that an epidemic broke out, and the plague did not pass from one man to another, but everyone who was killed by it got it straight from the air. In 1434 there were in Switzerland such quantities of hazel-nuts as no one had hitherto seen, thereupon there followed a rapid murderous plague, so that there was no place, however secluded in the mountains and valleys, in which at this time people were not carried off. In the year 1480 the rivers Tiber, Po, Danube, and others overflowed their banks so much that many people and cattle were drowned, and thereupon a plague ensued." To one chronicler the miraculous vision appears memorable " which in the year of Christ 1571 was seen at Cremnitz in the mountain towns of Hungary on Ascension Day in the evening to the great perturbation of all, when on the Schuelersberg there appeared so many black riders that the opinion was prevalent that the Turks were making a secret raid, but who rapidly disappeared again, and thereupon a raging plague broke out in the neighbourhood."

In the year 1680 there is reported in the so-called Journal : " That between Eisenberg and Dornberg thirty funeral biers all covered with black cloth were seen in broad daylight, among them on a bier a black man was standing with a white cross. When these had disappeared a great heat set in so that the people in this place could hardly stand it. But when the sun had set they perceived so sweet a perfume as if they were in a garden of roses. By this time they were all plunged in perturbation. Whereupon the epidemic set in in Thuringia in many places."

Not only before but during the plague signs and omens

appeared in multitudes. Thus in the fourteenth and fifteenth centuries it happened repeatedly that when bread was taken from the oven and cut some drops of blood fell out. " In the year 1501 small crosses, white, red, and the colour of blood and matter, fell on the women's veils and the clothes of the people, even on those that were stowed away in chests and drawers. In the following year such crosses fell upon the people and drops of blood were observed on the walls. Thereupon there ensued a great plague, and those on whom the crosses had fallen generally died." All those who in the previous year had seen the crosses and stains on their clothes were seized with despair, and having no hope, believing that they were bound to die, they awaited daily with fear and trembling the end of their lives, letting things go as they liked and taking no heed of anything.

In Mark Brandenburg no one tilled the fields any more, the gardens were neglected, the cattle were not tended, as everyone expected death the next moment. The bishops issued pastorals in which they announced the anger of God and instituted great festivals. "In the year 1599, when the great plague predicted by him had broken out, Johann Kepler wrote from Graz to his friend, Professor Mastlin, in Tuebingen that his little daughter, Susannah, had succumbed to the plague. " Should her father die very shortly it would not come unexpected to him. When a short time ago here and there in Hungary blood-red crosses appeared on the bodies of the people and other blood-red signs on the house-doors, walls, and benches, I was, as far as I know, the first in the town to perceive a little cross on my left foot, the colour of which merged from blood-red to yellow. It appeared on that part of the foot where the back spreads out, right in the middle between the root of the shin and the toes. I should think that this and no other was the place where the nail of the cross was driven into Christ's foot. In some people, as I am informed, there is a mark of a drop of blood on the surface of the hand. Christ's hands were also transfixed. But no one here has anything similar to that which I have."

As late as 1704, in various villages in the jurisdiction of Insterburg in East Prussia, markings of a similar nature were observed and considered to be Hebrew letters.

Not until a few decades later did a courageous natural scientist prove that the blood-stains were due to the excrements of butterflies (*leucoma dispar*). When the storm blast—and "it is not to be taken lightly and waved away"—prostrates the straightest and stoutest trees, and not only tears many branches from the finest trees, but also rips off the freshest fruit, it then seems to the Thuringian chronicler to be an omen that many young, strong and lusty people will be laid low and carried off by the plague. During the plague of 1565 in Italy rumblings of thunder were heard day and night, as in a war, together with the turmoil and noise as of a mighty army. In Germany in many places a noise was heard as if a hearse were passing through the streets of its own accord, "and as if other phantom gravediggers were meeting the real gravediggers on their return from the cemetery, as is frequently said to have happened to the gravediggers, the so-called wicked men of Leipzig, inspiring them with the greatest horror."

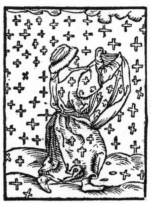

"CROSSES ON CLOTHES."
From Joh. Stumpff's Swiss Chronicle.

On the termination of the plague the spirits and apparitions generally developed particular activity—" as the wicked fiend then by the grace of God endeavoured to overthrow many more, and sought to attain one more and yet another." In the seventeenth century, particularly distinguished by its superstition, the newspapers already began greedily to collect items of news of this sensational nature. An example of the horror column of journalism of that period is a paper of September 1, 1682, entitled " Truthful and exact account of the native town of the late Dr. Luther—how Eisleben was nearly extinguished and has now recovered." The paper is of particular interest, as it was evidently written by an opponent of the Reformation : " Conditions in Eisleben are such as to break one's heart and bring tears into one's eyes, and would make one believe that God has forgone all mercy. It would be vain to endeavour to describe the great quantities of corpses. In Long Street all citizens with the exception of four are dead, the whole of Bell Street is exterminated with the exception of three. All the carpenters, brewers, turners, as well as fifteen bakers, together with their families, are dead. Many are as full of plague as Lazarus was of boils. The new town of Eisleben has been exterminated with the exception of twelve citizens. The cattle have died of starvation, decaying cattle fill the byres. The town of Merseburg dispatched five cattle men, but they were hardly able to endure it for five days on account of the fearful stench that has arisen; the surviving cattle have been driven into the Rapuse meadows. The town of Naumburg has sent five score of boards together with nails, victuals, and a hundred Rixdollars in cash. In the cemetery of Eisleben on the 6th inst. at night the following incident was noticed : When during the night the gravediggers were hard at work digging trenches, for on many days between eighty and ninety have died, they suddenly observed that the cemetery church, more especially the pulpit, was lighted up by bright sunshine. But on their going up to it so deep a darkness and black, thick fog came over the graveyard that they could hardly see one another, and which they took to be an evil omen. Thus day and night gruesome evil spirits are seen frightening the people, goblins grinning at them and pelting them, but also many white ghosts and spectres, so that it is assumed that the plague might abate. The plague poison is so virulent that in comparison the former plague was but mere child's play, as quite recently a citizen infected by the poison, on relapsing into an arm-chair, in the same moment swelled up and burst. The eyes of the dead as well as those of the still living infected persons are all burst asunder. Medicines are no longer of avail, nor does anyone desire to use any, as the infection poison has been found to be unconquerable. In short, nothing is heard in Eisleben but the weeping and wailing of those still alive, and the gibbering of the evil spirits, of the laughing goblins—so that every town and community should pray to merciful God for preservation. Wolferstedt, near Altstadt, has now been infected; in Mittelhausen, Enersdorf, Leuningen, Wallhausen, etc., the plague is raging. Also at Homborg, near Obervort, the inhabitants of the houses, with the exception of eight, have been exterminated; in Mertenriez all inhabitants with the exception of seven. In Manfeld and Leinbach, in the neighbourhood of Eisleben, the plague continues. At Hottstedt two whole streets have been exterminated. At Magdeburg things threaten to become as bad as at Eisleben. When Magister Hardte expired in his agony a blue smoke was seen to rise from his throat, and this in the presence of the dean; the same has been observed in the case of others expiring. In the same manner blue smoke has been observed to rise from the gables of houses at Eisleben all the inhabitants of which have died. In the church of St. Peter blue smoke has been observed high up near the ceiling; on this account the church is shunned, particularly as the parish has been exterminated."

In an indignant reply by an inhabitant of Eisleben to this horror-monger's report the following statements, among others, are made : " The statement in regard to Magister Hardte, a most truthful, honest and exemplary priest, is not surprising, nor that an attempt should be made to slander the honest man in his grave. Medical men can furnish reports concerning this to the effect that it is by no means unusual, but naturally takes place in the case of all expiring men. In the same manner the smoke must naturally rise through the gable if the kitchen fire is lighted and the chimney is defective."

In London during the plague of 1665 there appeared a host of sensational pamphlets all predicting the destruction of the town. Daniel Defoe mentions particularly " Lilly's Almanach." He also relates how many people were driven mad by such publications and rushed about the streets prophesying all kinds of horrors. The trade of soothsaying was carried on so commonly and openly that it was quite usual to find a sign above a door saying " Here lives a prophet, an astrologer, etc."

Sensible men like Adam von Lebenwald, in his " Town and Country Book of House Medicine," 1695, strongly opposes such wanton mischief which cost many a man his life : " Credence should not be given to every tramp, false prophet, and news reporter who of every black cloud construct a bier, of every so-called shooting-star a flying dragon or a comet, from the reflection of starlight foretell I know not what judgment and infliction, and in every fiery celestial phenomenon see an opening of the heavens, and who then in uneven rhymes chant these miracles to the populace, even causing lying sheets to be printed by which they inspire the simple with great fear and tribulation, but themselves reap a rich harvest of money; verily the devil and his accomplices can conjure up marvellous and deceptive phantasms and imaginations in the elements with which to render us pusillanimous and superstitious."

APPENDIX

As to whether Death sent certain Precursors to Vienna and warned of his Descent
(*Abraham a Santa-Clara*)

Before proceeding to describe in full detail the course of the fell disease, it would appear incumbent to know if no unusual signs and indications had preceded it from which an outbreak of the plague in Vienna might have been predicted. Such signs are commonly divided into four kinds—namely, in air, water, earth, and heavenly signs; to the heavenly signs belong sinister aspects and baneful constellations, as well as the miserable comets, which generally prove to be reliable precursors of the plague, as in the year 1618 a comet appeared after which plagues ensued in various places. In the year 1606 a comet was seen, after which a general plague traversed the world. In 1582 a comet brought so violent a plague upon Majo, Prague, Thuringia, the Netherlands, and other places that in Thuringia it carried off 37,000 and in the Netherlands 46,415. That at this time a comet appeared here no one with truth could maintain. But that this year there was from above a baneful conjunction of the stars was proved recently beyond all doubt by a well-known physician in a treatise. Regarding the air signs, they consist in variations of the weather in the different seasons, a prevalence of south wind, excess of rain, which in this year has been incessant; then evil smelling mists are blamed, as indicative of the plague, and of these, indeed, several were observed last autumn. In my opinion the plague is caused not only by the mists but by godless misters.

Water signs are generally sudden overflowing of the rivers, also when the wells turn muddy and brackish, also it is a sure sign when fish and crabs leave their water and holes and withdraw to the shores, also when frogs and toads are seen in great quantities.   But it is also certain that when fishy methods are used in the law courts and common decency assumes the crooked walk of the crab, and in all dark corners and taverns frivolous and shameless toads are to be found, that this will not tarry to send the plague.

Earth signs are unusual lack of fertility of the soil and failure of the crops of trees, the fields, and the vineyards, also

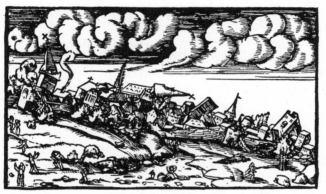

A GREAT EARTHQUAKE.
From Sebastian Muenster's " Cosmographia."

the earthquakes ; further when in the autumn the spring flowers and herbs once more grow green and flower, when the multitude of locusts, beetles, vineyard moths and mice devour the fruit of the earth everywhere.   It cannot be denied that this year there was a decided failure of the crops in Vienna, especially of the grain crops, but many more growths of fungus nature and the like have been found than in other years.   But it should be known that not only mice, but also wicked little human mice announce the approach of a plague.   Thus, too, when human ill weeds grow apace, sow thistles, goats' beards, and the like, you know well what is meant—all these are frequently precursors of a plague.

In addition there are other signs which generally precede

a plague, such as frequent meteors or shooting-stars. Thus in 1538 Swabia, Switzerland, and Bavaria sustained a plague together with an unheard-of outbreak of dysentery, and this is said to have been announced by shooting-stars. In the year 1536 shooting-stars of this kind were observed in Hungary in the form of a tongue, as if drawn with black pumice-stone. Around Vienna the common people, particularly the vineyard guards, swore on oath that at this time they frequently observed shooting-stars. To this category belongs what is heard at night-time—a weeping and wailing which by the credulous populace is called "the wail," but in the Salzburg district the common people call it "death and his wife"; experience shows that such things, any of them, announce an epidemic.

In the same manner it has been observed that when little children playing in the streets, in addition to riding on hobby horses and building houses, occasionally play at funerals and funeral processions, that such childish play has frequently been the prelude to a tragedy—a fact to which no definite cause can be attributed, but which is founded on experience. Of such occurrences nothing has been noted here, nor has any prophet arisen who predicted the coming evil, although the neighbouring kingdom of Hungary was so badly afflicted by this disease and assumed the rôle of a Sibylla; but omniscient God has by his indiscernible wisdom rendered such prophecies ridiculous among us, doubtless in order that his pure justice may take its course. Most curious is what is reported by some reliable men, according to whom a man in the hour of his death assured, on the earnest inquiry of his confessor and wishing it to be taken as his last dying testimony, that he together with another for certain business had proceeded to Hernals, the market borough nearest Vienna, and had tarried there somewhat late against his will; so that, overtaken by night, he had to make his way home in the dark, although the pale moon, at that time full, changed the night into bright day, and he could observe everything so clearly that he would even have undertaken to read a letter; then he heard—and he stood still a long time to listen, at a well-known spot in the fields—a mournful tune, sung as if many sad voices were mournfully intoning and repeating the following words " *Placebo Domino*

in regione Vivorum." Which words it is the custom of the
Catholic Church to sing at funerals; and, behold! not long afterwards the plague broke out and, unconscious of the fact, on the
very place where this mournful music had been heard a huge
burial trench was dug in which several thousands lie buried.
This music was heard by several others, but these were
ignorant of the Latin language and, therefore, could not understand the words. I do not entertain the least doubt about
this story and believe firmly that more signs of this nature
were vouchsafed, of which the people relate many which I did
not insert here, as in such matters untruths so easily slip in.
It is true our most kind God very frequently announces great
evils by certain precursory signs. And yet it should be no
little comfort that the above mentioned verse, " *Placebo
Domino,"* was heard sung by an invisible choir of the dead,
indicating that God the All Merciful had saved the majority
of the dead and compensated the shortening of their days on
earth by eternal life, as it was revealed in the year 1489 at
Brussels, when 35,000 people died of the plague, that all had
obtained salvation with the exception of two, one of whom
had doubted the boundless mercy of God, and the other
had voluntarily neglected confession and the sacrament of
repentance.

CHAPTER III

THE MEDICAL PROFESSION AND THE PLAGUE

The helplessness of the physicians—Medicine in the fetters of theology—
Ecclesiastic quacks—Astrology and medicine—Sorcery—Conscien-
tiousness of contemporary physicians—Development of anatomical
science—Rash healers—Successful doctors deprived of their gains
by municipalities—Senseless behaviour of population—Drunken
surgeons—German medical science—Paracelsus as impediment—
The theory of contagion—Heroes of modern medicine.

Appendix : Post-mortem report from the year 1713.

ON the whole the physicians were quite helpless in the face of
the plague. The most eminent among them confessed it
frankly. Chalin de Vinario declared : " Every pronounced
case of plague is incurable." And Guy de Chauliac, the
celebrated physician in ordinary to Clement VI, the father of
French surgery, in his principal work, *" La Grande Chirugie,"*
writes: "The disease was most humiliating for the physicians,
who were unable to render any assistance, all the more as, for
fear of infection, they did not venture to visit the patients,
and if they did could do no good and consequently earn no
fees, for all infected died with the exception of some towards
the end of the epidemic, who escaped, as the boils had been
able to mature." They therefore restricted themselves
mainly to prophylactic measures, and agreed with the Church
that the best and most efficacious preventive means was the
fear of God, " for by this the venomous astral arrows may be
averted."

To-day when, thanks to the immortal achievements of
Yersin and Koch, the bacteriological character of the plague
has been established, we can understand that even the highest
medical genius was capable of attaining very little. And just
at the period of the great plague epidemic medical science
inspired by the works of the Greeks, so hated by the Church,

which had just penetrated from the Orient to Italy, had developed so magnificently.

The circumstance that the universities were under the jurisdiction of the Church, in whose estimation it was a secondary science, " as its aim was only care of the body and not the mind," raised immense difficulties. In a small allegorical poem of the thirteenth century, " The Marriage of the Seven Arts and the Seven Virtues," Grammar, after having married her daughters Dialectic, Geometry, Music, Rhetoric, and Theology, and after having united herself with the priesthood, introduces Lady Physics (by which name medicine was then known, as we still speak of physicians) and begs that a husband be found for her too. But the new arrival has a very bad reception and is told: "You are not of our blood, we can give you no council." In a little anonymous primer for doctors of the period we find that it was the first duty of the physician on entering the house to ask the relations of the patient if he had confessed and received the holy sacrament, as upon this in the first instance his salvation depended. For this he had to use the following locution : " The soul is more worthy than the body, therefore its salvation goeth before all things." The patient must in the name of God be induced to seek the salvation of his soul, and if he has not yet done so, he must do it at once or promise to do it, for most frequently sickness is the consequence of our sins. Thus the enlightened physician was obliged to play a double rôle in accordance with the prevailing opinions of the time—indeed in the twelfth and thirteenth centuries he had to unite the ecclesiastic profession with medical science so as to escape the envy and persecution of the clergy. It did not suit the Church that men enlightened by the knowledge of natural science should enjoy the intimacy of princes and the great men of the country. " The priests pushed and crowded round the sick beds and endeavoured to prove the efficiency of their appeals to the saints, their intercessions and relics, their consecrated candles, masses, endowment vows, sacrifices and other pious means of robbery. If a physician attained a good cure, it was attributed to the intercession of the saints, the vows or the prayers of the priests. If the cure was a failure, the physicians were rendered responsible for the death of the patient, and the lack of trust in God and the saints was stated to be the cause of death, which was regarded as a punishment of God, for which the relations had to do penance by an excess of masses for the repose of the soul." Right into the eighteenth century the science of medicine had to hold her own against ecclesiastic encroachments, and was to some extent still encumbered by theological prejudice. A witty doctor, Christian Diderich, was impelled to make the following statement as late as 1710 : " An honest medical man can as little be an atheist as an angel can be a devil, as both in his studies as in his practice he has the great works of God before his eyes. But as a medical man he leaves this side to those by whom the holy ghost pronounces a judgment against the mockers of ecclesiastic teachers with the words : If any man rely on having Christ, let him think with himself that as he has Christ we too have Christ. As, on the other hand, no sensible theologian converts his church into an apothecary where may be obtained theriac, electuria, panacæ, ointments, Balsam sulphuris, clyster, and the like."

The necessary connection with theology endowed all mediæval medicine with the character of quackery, against which minds like Petrarch and Gerson inveighed so sarcastically. It must be admitted that even the most enlightened minds were swayed by astrology and magic, which occupy a prominent place in the opinions of medical faculties of that period, of which the opinion of the Paris faculty that was drawn up by order of the king Philip of Valois in 1348 is the best known. The influence of astrology on medicine attained its climax in the sixteenth and seventeenth centuries. Physics and chemistry at that period throughout Europe taught in an occult manner, nearly as if they had been magic. If one turns to the works of Albertus Magnus it is difficult to determine where the language of simile begins and where it ends. In Italy Peter of Apone maintained that he had been instructed in the seven free arts by seven spirits which he had conjured into a crystal. All money that he spent returned to his pocket (this may be easily believed, as this physician charged 150 lires for every visit paid outside the town and demanded 400 ducats a day from the sick Pope Honorius IV). In fact, most people were incapable of understanding his symbolic language and ideas, and he was to be seized by the

Inquisition when, fortunately for him, he died, whereupon his effigy was burnt and his corpse secretly buried by his mistress.

Among the people the physicians were extremely unpopular, and only on the rarest occasions did they apply to them, as was the case with most princes, preferring alchemists, magicians and quacks, of whom there were multitudes :

> Monks, parsons, and chemists, dentists and shavers,
> Quacks and greasers and all kinds of bathers,
> Jews and with wisdom ninefold endowed wives,
> They cure with their rubbish all the ills of our lives.

As the plague was immediately recognised as a contagious disease by the medical authorities of the fourteenth century, most physicians refused to attend the sufferers, whereas the avarice of the quacks was deterred by no danger. Guy de Chauliac confesses that he only remained at his post for fear of disgrace. And Chalin de Vinario praises the doctors, who sought safety with a cynicism which gives a poor impression of the sense of duty of the profession. " As to approach the patients is coupled with certain danger," he writes, " there are but few physicians who for an enormous fee expose themselves to so great a peril. In my opinion they are quite right, for many who were not prudent enough to hold back have been involved in the fate of their patients. No one is so blind and senseless that he should care more for the salvation of others than for his own, particularly in the case of so infectious a disease." This maxim Vinario certainly did not apply to himself, but staked his own life. Chauliac overcame a severe attack of the plague, as he relates himself, and then in 1363 succumbed to a second infection. Gentilis de Fulgineo of Perugia, a professor of medicine celebrated throughout Italy, war carried off by the plague, a victim to his duty, in 1348. Under his auspices the corpses of plague victims were dissected several times at Perugia. What the medical men believed to have discovered was a small boil in the vicinity of the heart filled with poison, and they attributed the miserable death of young and old to the poisoning of the blood by secretions from this boil. Anatomy was the youngest and most hopeful branch of medical science of the period. The Council of Tours in 1163 had still prohibited the shedding of blood, i.e. to engage in

surgical practice. *Ecclesia abhorret a sanguine.* Emperor
Frederick II was the first to permit the dissection of the
human body in his empire and to establish a chair of anatomy.
It is to him and Charles VI of France, who issued a decree
ordering that every year the corpse of some executed criminal
should be handed over to the medical faculty of Montpelier,
to this we owe the foundation of a scientific doctrine of the
diseases of the human body. At Vienna the celebrated
physician, Marsilius Galleati of Padua, introduced anatomy as

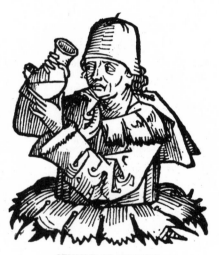

GENTILE DI FOLIGNO.
From Schedel's Chronicle.

a subject of medical instruction in 1404. The celebrated
Viennese physician Sorbait, who succeeded in healing some
hundreds in the hospital, overcame the plague twice, in 1665
and 1680. It is related of Heinrico Sayer that in 1665, when
the plague was raging in England, he fearlessly attended all
patients rich and poor, daily administered their medicine, and
with his own hands bound up their boils, plague glands, and
spots, thus saving the life of many. In this dangerous occu-
pation he availed himself of no other means of preservation
than to take a long draught of good strong wine before entering the houses of those infected; then he set about his work

with his patients and repeated the same means on its completion ; in this manner he preserved himself a long time. " But one must not be too bold and venturesome," the chronicler continues, " nor undertake too much, lest one should meet with the same fate as this same medical man. For after having moved about in the midst of the plague for a long time and waited on his patients as if the plague could not assail him, he was requested as a second Aesculapius to repair to another place, where the plague was still more virulent ; there he was soon seized by the plague when he ventured at the house of a great lord, with whom he was intimate and who was suffering from the plague, to sleep with him in the same bed, and as the arts which had saved all others were of no avail to their master and possessor, to the great sorrow and distress of many, was carried off by the disease."

In nearly all countries there was a repetition of what Rolandus Capellutus Chrysopolitanus relates of the epidemic of Parma in the year 1468 : " When the epidemic of plague had abated the medical men and physicians who had attended the patients were arrested by the authorities and thrown into the prisons, being accused of all kinds of murders and manslaughter, and frequently the money which the medical men had acquired with great exertion and work and with extreme danger to their lives was taken from them by force." That it could be dangerous to be too successful in curing is shown by the example of the physician Marquier, who in 1601, at Saint-Lo in Normandy, was accused of magic because he had healed more sufferers than his colleagues and had saved too many from the plague. He appealed to the recognised authority and prescriptions of his teacher, the surgeon Ambroise Paré, but without avail, for after a six-day trial he was banished from Saint-Lo together with his daughter. At the beginning of the plague the people, particularly in Italy, were frequently of opinion that the doctors themselves caused the rumour of the outbreak to be circulated so as to induce the population to resort to them. A conception to which the aged, venerable Ludovico Settala, one of the leading physicians and philosophers of Milan, nearly fell victim in 1630. On his return from his patients he was suddenly surrounded by hordes of porters and market women, who howled at him that he was the principal physician and original instigator of those who with stick and beard were spreading terror throughout the town. Only the courage of the litter-bearers, who were devoted to him and carried him to the house of a friend, saved him from being lynched by the raving rabble. In all countries we meet in times of plague with complaints of the doctors of the obstinacy of the patients. The surgeon of the administrative district of Szabin in East Prussia applied in 1710 to be recalled, as all medical assistance was useless. The surviving remnant of the population had fled to the woods and were hopelessly abandoned to their fate. The only remaining peasant obstinately refused to take any medicine, and it was useless to incur further expenses for the prescribed treatment. " The incredible lack of obedience," he continues his report, " prevents all benefit to those still alive. With all due submission I, therefore, inquire if an example should not be made of some or the others of them, particularly as the usual Lithuanian form of chastisement by the public executioner is of no avail." The judicial authorities of the district had on July 26, 1710, an edict read from the pulpits threatening that all those would be regarded as suicides and that their corpses would be publicly hanged who refused to take the prescribed medicines, even if these should prove to be of no avail. In the same manner the Prussian Sanitary Commission had submitted a resolution to the King that gallows should be erected for those who refused to take their concoctions, and that they should be hanged on them in their coffins. There is an interesting report of July 25, 1710, from the district of Insterburg containing complaints about the famous, well-known member of the Koenigsberg Sanitary Commission, Professor Dr. Emmerich, as well as about Dr. Rossler, who were on a tour of inspection in Lithuania. The report states : " Although the cures undertaken by the surgeons are accompanied by so little success, this would seem to cause them little anxiety, as with the help of strong Insterburg ale they spend their time in joy and merriment; thus, to give a particular instance, they spent the night of June 16th–17th at the house of Sergeant Forstmann with drinking, dancing, and carousing. But that was not all: they were seen at 4 a.m. in full daylight with a band of music, and thereupon, without changing their clothes or lying down, they repaired to the house of Apothecary Hering, their ordinary quarters, for breakfast, and continued their drinking throughout the day until finally, towards the evening of the 17th, they drove from Insterburg to Goldap, and then further to Stallupoenen and Ragnit in company of the sheriff, during which journey, as their companion took them a somewhat circuitous route, there was no lack of merriment and drinking. But in spite of this the doctors were not drunk but only merry, and it would appear that this commission trip was by no means disagreeable to them, as up to the present all three have not returned."

Inquiry into the particular merits of medical science in Germany reveals the undeniable fact that it was far behind that of the French, and particularly of the Italians, on which in the fourteenth century it was entirely dependent. However great physicians there were in subsequent centuries— such men as Wierus, Plattner, Gessner, Krato—they lacked the sane liberal outlook which distinguished particularly the Italians. By a pursuit of the phantoms of the " reformer " of Einsiedeln, Theophrastus Bombastus Paracelsus, the true line of development in medical science was lost, and extremely laborious and painful by-paths had to be trodden before it was possible to pick it up again. The magic therapeutics of Paracelsus, which were further developed by his ingenious successors von Helmont and Robert Flood, were based on the conception that a common original force, termed *Magnale Magnum*, or Universal Soul, connected all bodies with one another. "Every body possesses a peculiar essence, a particular spirit by means of which it exerts an influence on bodies related to it and cause modifications in their state of health ; he who is familiar with these spirits will prove a good physician. They are frequently recognisable by signature, certain external signs which coincide with their spirit. The sympathetic healing process is accomplished by magnetic force, stimulated to a higher degree of activity, reacting on the body in whose circle of vitality it is situated, and again stimulating the vital force of this body to an activity capable of expulsing the disease, or by itself attracting the disease and thus ridding the body of it. The activity of these magnetic forces hidden in the vital spirit is mainly determined by the essence of materials brought into contact with it. The Paracelsists were at great pains to procure magnets of this description which, on the one hand, stimulated the vital spirit in human beings, and, on the other, were supposed to attract diseases and, as it was believed that the vital spirit still adhered to human blood and human excrements, magnets were made consisting of the materials which, in the opinion of the time, were the most filthy imaginable. Paracelsus called these material bases of the spirit, mummies. The development of the forces within the mummy is generally effected by means of putrefaction—a process carried out in various manners. Thus, for instance, to convert blood into a mummy it was extracted from a healthy human subject, and let into an eggshell; the egg was firmly closed with isinglass and placed under a sitting hen till the chickens were hatched from the other eggs. A carneous mass is then found in the egg; this is placed in the bake-oven till the bread is baked, and is kept for use." This mummy taken from a healthy subject develops magnetic forces, taken from a diseased subject it serves to cure all diseases ; for if the mummy is applied to the diseased limb so that it is mingled with its sweat, if given to eat to any animal or grafted into any tree, the most obdurate diseases may be overcome.

Most of the repulsive cures of which we shall treat in the next chapter can be traced back to the magic treatment and organic therapeutics of Paracelsus. The baneful influence of the reformer also retarded progress in other countries, even in Italy, and sapped the beneficial effect of the theory of contagion as developed in 1540 by Nicolaus Massa and subsequently by Victor Bonagentibus.

A decisive victory for the theory of contagion was first obtained by the work of Marsaria in 1577–78 during the plague of Vicenza. His theory concerning contagion and importation of the plague caused the authorities of Vicenza to institute a whole system of sanitary measures, and was evidently the cause that at Vicenza the plague passed over much more rapidly and with less serious consequences than in other Italian towns. Of extreme interest are the first inklings of the bacterial origin of the plague. The Jesuit Father, Athanasius Kircher, of Fulda, was of opinion—as we read in the treatise on the plague by Johannes Amerianos in 1667

—that he had discovered something peculiar and got to the bottom of the matter : " Thus, he writes that the plague is nothing but a multitude of small animals and diminutive worms which fly about in the air, and when drawn into the body by the action of breathing they vitiate the blood, impair the spirits, and finally gnaw into the flesh and glands. When they fly from an infected body, or, in some other manner, are received by a healthy subject, the plague is spread by them. Protection against them could be attained by lighting large and flaming fires by means of which their wings, feet, or probosces, etc., are burnt off, so that they can no longer fly about and vitiate the blood of human beings and gnaw their bodies." By means of magnifying glasses he had observed that the air was full of worms, and by various experiments he proved that decaying matter produced worms and described accurately how the experiment was carried out, and that they could then be seen under the microscope. "But," he added, "it must not be believed that any usual microscope will serve ; it must be like mine, which enlarges a thousandfold." Johann Georg Nicolai Dietrich (1714) expresses his opinion in regard to Kircher's " little plague worms " as follows : " To confess the truth it seems to me that the learned man wished to bequeath to posterity a satyrical history of the plague and to ridicule the method of Hippocrates, who for this purpose fired whole forests in order to burn the wings of the plague insects flying about in the air." Antrechau, who distinguished himself during the plague at Toulon in 1721, on the other hand, supported Kircher's view. His book was translated into German by Knigge in 1794, and in a preface Reimarus expresses himself as follows : " Who can fathom the limits of life in nature ? Cannot still more minute (I hardly dare to call them animals) exist which in their composition and conditions of life vary as much from the infusoria as these from all animals previously known ? The suggestion is offered by the fact that these appear to be pursuing something still more minute which is no longer revealed by the magnifying glass." In the year 1720 Eggerdes got very near the truth. " If now the plague is attributable to such material poisonous entities which are transferred in a continuous chain from one place to another, then this poison must be of such a nature that it is capable of reproducing itself *ad infinitum.*"

In the plague treatise of Conrad Berthold Behrends (1714) the surmise is expressed that the contagious matter is contained exclusively in the air surrounding every patient.

Of further interest is the predisposition theory expounded by Theodosius Tabernomontanus in his plague treatise in 1582. " This disease," he writes, " is pernicious to blood relatives and all of the same family. For so soon as one among relations is attacked by the disease it generally affects all other relations. And this because their bodies are predisposed to receive poison of such a nature, and this on account of the similarity of their physical constitution which they have inherited from birth and from their origin from the same seed. It is an everyday experience that if the plague lays hold of a family it is reluctant to leave it. And although members may not be living together in one town or place, and although the plague may have abated and returned after an interval of one year, two or three years, it starts again in such a family and carries off a few, so that it occasionally happens that a whole family is exterminated in the course of ten or twenty years, as experience has often proved."

Finally, we must mention the physicians of the nineteenth century whose names will remain immortal throughout all times. The first of them was Desgenettes (1762–1837), physician-in-chief to Napoleon's Orient Army, which in Egypt was decimated by a terrible attack of plague. When fear and horror threatened to destroy the *moral* of the army, Desgenettes, with the same courage displayed by Napoleon, when in the plague hospital at Jaffe he touched the plague sufferers and the corpses of those dead of the plague, gave an example of heroic devotion by making injections of pus taken from plague boils in his groins and under his armpits in the presence of the soldiers. This bold action appeased the men and facilitated the treatment of the sick. A second inoculation, still more terrible than the first, and which made all standing round grow pale, was carried out under the following circumstances : A dying plague patient besought Desgenettes, who was treating him, to share the rest of the medicine which had been prescribed for him. Without hesitation Desgenettes seized the glass of the patient and emptied it at a single draught.

The real victories over the plague are connected with the names of Pasteur, Koch, Roux, Behring, Kitasao, and Yersin. Pasteur in Paris and Koch in Berlin were the first to establish the bacterial character of infectious diseases. Roux discovered the toxins, the products from the transmutation of matter in the microbes. The Japanese Kitasao and the Frenchman Yersin, a pupil of Pasteur, discovered in 1894 at Hong-Kong, where a terrible epidemic of plague was raging, simultaneously and independently of one another the bacillus of the plague. Yersin also prepared a plague serum, and could boast that with this serum he had healed twenty-five out of twenty-eight patients. As a touching victim of devotion to duty, H. F. Mueller, a member of the Austrian Plague Commission, died at Vienna of pneumonic plague which he had contracted in the treatment of an attendant who had been infected in the laboratory after he had seen, treated, and dissected thousands of plague patients in India.

APPENDIX

Post-mortem Report of the Year 1713

Your Honours,

It being resolved to elucidate more fully the present Austrian epidemic which has caused so much trouble by means of an intrepid opening of a number of infected corpses, we yester morn at four o'clock hurried to the hospital well provided with all necessaries, and after having found there two rows of corpses, we halted between the churchyard and the corpse cart, and after having suffered considerably from the stench, we selected the following corpses.

I

A woman of the middle class hailing from the Contumatz neighbourhood, of vigorous age, with whitish hair, staring eyes, and gaping lips, the whole appearance terrible and menacing ; the tongue was protruding from the mouth, it was of a blackish colour. On the body there were neither boils nor carbuncles to be found, nor was it marked with any spots except on the left cheek, where here and there green spots or small markings were revealed, of which some larger ones, but of a red colour, were close to the ear. These spots were only on the skin and did not reach further, as was proved by the lancet. On opening the abdomen, we found the midriff quite normal and uninjured ; the stomach was not excessively distended by the swollen veins, but the lower orifice of the stomach as well as the duodenum were quite discoloured by green gall, the other intestines were quite normal except that the ileum was speckled. The large intestine was quite empty, and from the spleen to the rectum much wrinkled and contracted. The liver was quite shrivelled ; the gall bladder was filled with green gall ; the spleen was discoloured ; the kidneys were hard and shrivelled ; the uterus contracted and the bladder void of urine ; the uterus was quite natural ; the lungs, either from birth or on account of disease, had become firmly attached to the pleura on the right side. There is nothing to report in regard to the pericardium and pericardial fluid, although the heart appeared shrunken, the right and left ventricles were fouled with polypous blood and glutinous matter resembling black sticky tar, the pleura and peritoneum were healthy ; and after we had removed the top of the skull with a saw, the dura mater was found to be healthy, but the bloodvessels of the pia mater were much stained with blood similar to that in the heart ; the whole brain and the medulla spinali was collapsed and, like the heart, quite shrivelled. This in respect to the corpse from outside the town.

II

We now proceed to the body from the town.

An innkeeper with the constitution of a prize-fighter, marked on both shoulders and in the middle of the chest and all over the face with black stripes ; the opening of the skin revealed the subcutaneous fat and the deep fascia. Among the glands of the right groin was a terrible boil, which on pressure at its roots swelled so greatly that we examined it

more closely and found that it extended to the psoas muscle ;
it contained no mature matter, although already somewhat
putrid, so that it had infected the whole boil and all con-
tiguous parts. The base was marked by a large carbuncle,
the spread of which had affected all the membranes as far as
the sinews and surrounding veins, which were unaffected.
The stomach was very greatly distended, and internally
covered with black spots, the pancreas was normal, and the
duodenum full of green gall. The liver appeared quite
shrivelled and slippery ; the gall bladder was full of a blackish
green gall ; the spleen in better case. The large and small
intestines were found to be full of black stripes in the neighbourhood of the spleen and were quite putrid and decayed ;
the peritoneum revealed nothing remarkable ; the kidneys
were in a similar condition to the liver, the bladder full of
urine similar to vomited wine. In the right pleural cavity
we found water resembling green gall, which water or effusion
in the left pleural cavity between the lungs and pleura had
formed a thick membrane. The pleura and mediastinum as
well as the pericardium, but not the pericardial fluid, appeared
satisfactory. The heart was quite shrunken, both ventricles
being full of blood which was not thick, stagnant, curdled, or
mucous, as in the former case, but quite pure and liquid. In
the case of the first corpse, we did not need to fear that blood
flowing from the opened veins would impede us in our work,
but in this corpse the blood was quite liquid and thin.

III

A patient who died in the hospital had in the right groin
beside the abdomen a boil ; its roots extended into the cavity
of the abdomen, but it contained no matter. The intestines,
liver and spleen were shrivelled, the stomach was, so to say,
internally peeled, the peritoneum and pancreas were normal,
the lungs normal, the heart, as in the former cases, quite
shrunken, in the ventricles, however, we found the blood pure
and liquid.

And this we desire to submit to the honourable College of
Medicine, that they might the better be enabled to penetrate
and determine the present state and peculiarities of the

disease. It should further be pointed out that our lancets, although subjected to the usual thorough cleansing, have assumed a bluish colouring, as if they had been dipped in strong acid.

The most humble servants of the Honourable College of Medicine,

VALENTIN GORGIAS, *Phlac. et Medicinæ Doctor.*
FRANTZ ANTONI FUX, *Barber.*

Vienna in Austria, the 8th of July, 1713.

CHAPTER IV

PLAGUE REMEDIES

As in most cases the disease terminated with death and all
medical aid was of no avail, the protection of the healthy
appeared of greater importance than the treatment of the
sick. The first rule, which was obeyed not only by the rich
but also by large numbers of the poor, was flight. In nearly
all books on the plague we find mentioned the " three adverb
pills " of the Arabian physician Rhasis :

> Three little words the plague dispel,
> Quick, far and late, where'er you dwell.
> Start quick, go far and right away
> And with return till late delay.

or

> Three things by which each simple man
> From plague escape and sickness can,
> Start soon, flee far from town or land
> On which the plague has laid its hand,
> Return but late to such a place
> Where pestilence has stayed its pace.

For many the emptiness and depopulation of the large
towns was the most uncanny part of the whole plague. Thus
it is reported that in 1665 London looked like a desert. The
King and Queen had gone with the whole court to the West,
to uninfected places in the country; the High Councils and
High Court of Justice had been transferred. Parliament,

which had just been opened, had moved to Oxford. All rich
people with very few exceptions had left the town. The
stoppage of industry increased the misery and confusion.
Daniel Defoe makes a list of the classes particularly affected
by the lack of employment :

" (1) All master workmen in manufactures ; especially
such as belonged to ornament and the less necessary part of
the peoples' dress, clothes, and furniture for houses ; such as
ribband weavers and other weavers, gold and silver lace
makers, and gold and silver wire drawers, semptresses,
milliners, shoemakers, hatmakers, and glove-makers ; also
upholsterers, joiners, cabinet-makers, looking-glass-makers,
and innumerable trades which depend upon such as these. I
say the master workmen in such stopped their work, dismissed
their journeymen and workmen and all their dependents.

" (2) As merchandizing was at a full stop (for very few ships
ventured to come up the river and none at all went out), so all
the extraordinary officers of the Customs, likewise the watermen, carmen, porters, and all the poor whose labour depended
upon the merchants, were at once dismissed and put out of
business.

" (3) All the tradesmen usually employed in building or
repairing of houses were at a full stop, for the people were far
from wanting to build houses when so many thousand houses
were at once stript of their inhabitants ; so that this one
article turned out all ordinary workmen of that kind of
business, such as bricklayers, masons, carpenters, joiners,
plasterers, painters, glaziers, smiths, plumbers, and all the
labourers depending on such.

" (4) As navigation was at a stop, our ships neither coming
in nor going out as before, so the seamen were all out of employment, and many of them in the last and lowest degree of
distress ; and with the seamen were all the several tradesmen
and workmen belonging to and depending upon the building
and fitting out of ships ; such as ship carpenters, calkers,
rope-makers, dry-coopers, sail-makers, anchor smiths and
other smiths ; blockmakers, carvers, gunsmiths, ship chandlers,
ship carvers, and the like. The masters of those, perhaps,
might live upon their substance, but the traders were

universally at a stop, and consequently all their workmen discharged. Add to these that the river was in a manner without boats, and all or most part of the watermen, lightermen, boat builders, and lighter builders, in like manner idle, and laid by.

"(5) As all families, both those who fled and those who remained, reduced their standard of living, an innumerable quantity of lackeys, servants, shopkeepers, journeymen, commercial clerks, and such like people, particularly poor servant girls, were dismissed and remained friendless and helpless without work or lodging."

It was natural that princes were the first to flee from the plague. When in 1414 the plague was raging at Dijon, Duchess Margaret of Bavaria fled to Auxonne. But this was not far enough to appease her anxiety, and on August 28, 1414, she addressed the following lines to the authorities of the town of Dijon :

"DEAR AND MUCH BELOVED,
        "As at the present time plague and an epidemic of death are raging at Dijon and, as is well known to you, it is a question of a most infectious disease, it is our will and order that you should in good words make known to the inhabitants of the town of Dijon that none of them should presume to come to Auxonne, to which place we together with our children have repaired to escape the plague."

A fine proof of his paternal love of his people is supplied also by Louis XI. When in the year 1479 the plague broke out in Auxerre, to which place the King was in the habit of making a yearly pilgrimage to the tomb of Saint-Edmund, he on this occasion only sent his royal greetings to the Chapter of the Cathedral, but at the same time promised the holy brothers several vineyards at Dijon as a present on condition that they should pray to God, to the Holy Virgin, and to Saint-Edmund for him, the Dauphin, his son, and for the queen ! " And let prayers be said for the good digestion of our stomachs and that neither wine nor meat may cause us indigestion and that we may be preserved in good health."

Of the preventive and protective measures prescribed by the physicians I will first enumerate those recommended by the medical faculty of Paris in their report of October 1348 : "No poultry should be eaten, no waterfowl, no sucking pig, no old beef, altogether no fat meat. The meat of animals of a warm, dry constitution should be eaten, but no heating or irritating meat. We recommend broths with ground pepper, cinnamon, and spices, particularly to such people who eat little but choice food. It is injurious to sleep during the daytime. Sleep should not be extended beyond dawn or very little beyond it. Very little should be drunk at breakfast, lunch should be taken at 11 o'clock, and a little more wine may be drunk than at breakfast and the drink should be a clear, light wine mixed with one-sixth water. Dried or fresh fruit is innoxious if eaten together with wine. Without wine it may be dangerous. Beetroot and other fresh or preserved vegetables may prove injurious; spicy herbs such as sage and rosemary are, on the other hand, wholesome. Cold, moist, and watery foods are generally harmful. It is dangerous to go out at night till three in the morning on account of the dew. Fish should not be eaten, too much exercise may be injurious; the clothing should be warm, giving protection from cold, damp and rain, and nothing should be cooked in rain-water. With the meals a little treacle (*theriaca*) should be taken ; olive oil with food is mortal. Fat people should expose themselves to the sun. Excess of abstinence, excitement, anger, and drunkenness are dangerous. Diarrhœa is serious. Bathing dangerous. The bowels should be kept open by a clyster. Intercourse with women is mortal; there should be no coition nor should one sleep in any woman's bed."

The Italian physicians, e.g. Marsilio and Garbo, favoured epicurean precepts : " In the first instance no man should think of death ; nor should he conceive any passion for any man. Nothing should distress him, but all his thoughts should be directed to pleasing, agreeable and delicious things. Social intercourse should be avoided. Beautiful landscapes, fine gardens should be visited, particularly when odiferous plants are flowering, and best when the vines are in flower. But it should be avoided to tarry too long in the gardens, as the air is much more dangerous at night. In times of plague

light women should be entirely dispensed with as well as all
intercourse with drunkards. Thirst should not be suffered,
but only temperate drinking indulged in. Listening to beautiful, melodious songs is wholesome, as is also to enjoy the joys
of the fine season in the company of agreeable people. The
contemplation of gold and silver and other precious stones is
comforting to the heart."

A German physician, Jobus Lincelius of Zwickau, evidently
belongs to the Italian school, as he prescribes : " All physical
exertions and emotions of the mind should be avoided, such as
running, jumping, jealousy, anger, hatred, sadness, horror or
fear, licentiousness and the like, and those who, by the grace
of God, are in a position to do so, may spend their time in
relating tales and stories and with good music to delight their
hearts, as music was given to man by God to praise God and
give pleasure to mankind."

Serenity and light-heartedness were considered by the
physicians as particularly important, as they believed they
had observed that many had in some magic way taken the
plague in consequence of fear and horror. " Not the smallest
preservation in these *Morbis Popularibus* is not to be afraid,
and one should not imagine that one had the disease and not
paint the devil on the wall. For as soon as the fear of death
and imagination obtain the upper hand, then certainly what
we dread will occur." Therefore all such fears and thoughts
should be set aside entirely, or, as Paracelsus says, imagination loves to adhere to its own pitch and may easily be set
alight. As an example of the power of imagination the
unsatisfied craving of pregnant women is constantly quoted,
" who, when inspired by a great desire to eat a certain thing on
which they dwell in their imagination and which, if refused
them suddenly or is unable to be obtained, there appear upon
the child at its birth signs and marks of this same thing, due
only to the strong imagination of the woman, as is known to
many, and marks of this nature remain with the children for
their whole lives. Now if this lively imagination of the
pregnant woman can impress such marks on the child in the
womb, how much more can strong imaginations effect our own
bodies, as the body is ruled by the soul, in which such imagination originates." It is, therefore, important to believe firmly

that one cannot be affected by illness, for by such belief the
Archæus or *Aura vitalis* is fortified, i.e. the idea which is
opposed to the pernicious idea which might be inspired in us
by fear and dread.   All physicians for that reason recommend
wine as a " care-lifter."   " But in such times all wine-bibbers
and children of Bacchus, who spend day and night in the service
of their father, should be wary."   A proverb says : " Neither
drunk nor yet too sober in times of plague is the way to get
over," and Hans Folz, the Mastersinger, writes :

> And in your mind this warning hold,
> Have wine that's strong and clear and old,
> Wash every morning with it clear
> Hands, mouth and face and nose and ear,
> Shoulders and body everywhere,
> And drink a sup with morning fare
> To raise the heart and purge the blood,
> Thus many have the plague withstood.

The knight Hans von Schweinichen relates in the story of
his life how, during the great plague at Cologne in 1576, he
never yielded to fear but trusted in God, for he was sure that
he would not die.   But every morning on rising he had " a
little vinegar of wine with toasted bread together with his
breakfast, and followed it up with a copious draught of wine.
Thus God preserved him and his master's servants so that not
a single one of them died."   As the plague generally abated
in October, its decrease on the Rhine was attributed to the
new wine.

That Clement VI should have sat between two huge fires
during the plague does not strike us, who know how little
capable the plague bacillus is of resisting heat, as foolish.
But the mad fumigating for the purpose of cleansing the air
from the plague poison was of little use.   They burnt incense,
juniper shrubs and berries, laurel leaves, fir-wood, cypress and
pine, beech and aloe, lemon and orange leaves, oak leaves,
wormwood, balm mint, rosemary, thyme, green rue, amber,
mastic, laudanum, storax, birchbark, red myrrh, sage, lavender, majoram, camphor, sulphur.   The fumigations were so
intensive that canaries were suffocated in the rooms, sparrows
fell from the roofs and the young swallows died in their nests
and the old ones flew away.   The common people attributed

the dying of the birds to infection in the air—Helmont claimed to have observed that in the Alps the clouds which he could touch with his hand stank—and the plague doctor Diderich (1713) was only able to cure the plague missionary of this erroneous conception by making beneath a swallow's nest on a house a big fumigating fire with the usual poisonous fumes, on which the old birds flew away and the young ones were soon found to be dead in the nest. Another method of purifying the air was the use of essences and aromatic oils of various kinds of herbs, which were made to evaporate on glowing bricks. The whole house was also rubbed down with them, and they were poured on pocket-handkerchiefs so that they

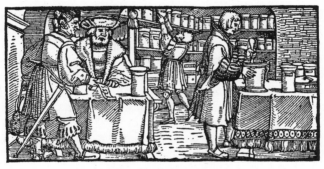

MEDIÆVAL APOTHECARY.
From the " Pestregiment " of Quintorius Joannes.

might be inhaled in the streets. The plague water and essences gave the initiative for the invention of Eau de Cologne, which was first prepared by the Italian, Johann Maria Farina, about 1700 at Cologne. An idea of the business done by doctors and apothecaries may be formed by reading the following arrangements for a week :

To be held under the nose on going out and inhaled.

Sunday : In the apothecaries I have prescribed an essence consisting of rue, roses, cloves, juniper, etc., with which a clean sponge may be impregnated, and this placed in a small box made of silver or juniper, aloe, sandal or rose wood, and held at the nose ; instead of this essence a few drops of amber, juniper oil, etc., may be poured on the sponge. *Monday :* Scent boxes for men and women will be ready containing green rue, wormwood, rosemary, majoram, poley and thyme. *Tuesday:* Valerian, alant, juniper, soaked in vinegar, juniper berries. *Wednesday:* Juniper, lavender, or angelica oil to be poured on a sponge ; red fern, milfoil, lavender, roses. *Thursday:* Paradise or sandal wood, pomander, black softened cumin, coriander, myrrh and incense. *Friday:* Orange and lemon peel, cloves, mace, each separate or mixed together with a little saffron poured on a rag and moistened with essence of roses or cloves. *Saturday:* Valerian, wormseed, angelica, either alone or mixed with other essences, benzoin, styrax calamita, civet thiesem, pomander, etc.

The scent apple (*Pomus ambræ*) is to be seen in numerous woodcuts of the sixteenth century, and in portraits, particularly of royal personages, of the sixteenth and seventeenth centuries. It has only quite recently been recognised as a protective against the plague. In Holland and England tobacco was regarded as a particularly efficacious means of protection. To the present day the Dutch anti-plague pipes of the year 1665 are preserved in the South Kensington Museum. It was not till this period that Dutch clay pipes, as Sticker relates, spread through Westphalia to the Rhineland. Snuff was also regarded as an efficacious protection. " Reason, because in infectious places the poisonous atoms fly about, and if they are caught in the nose they penetrate the body and may easily cause inflammation, therefore snuff should be used that they may be expelled at once." The Berlin municipal medical officer, Fleck, in his treatise on the plague in 1556, exhorts his readers to pay special attention to the cleansing of mouth, teeth, and nose ; he recommends several mouth washes, tooth powders, and tooth-picks. The protective measures adopted by many doctors in the large towns produced a very amusing effect. The " Beak Doctors," by their fantastic disguise, cheered the patients and were the terror of the children in the streets :

As may be seen on picture here,
In Rome the doctors do appear,
When to their patients they are called,
In places by the plague appalled,
Their hats and cloaks, of fashion new,
Are made of oilcloth, dark of hue,

Their caps with glasses are designed,
Their bills with antidotes all lined,
That foulsome air may do no harm,
Nor cause the doctor man alarm
The staff in hand must serve to show
Their noble trade where'er they go.

As the opinion prevailed that the air was, so to say, stiff in times of plague, it was deemed necessary to set it in motion artificially and break it up. For this purpose all bells were rung; cannons, muskets, and blunderbusses were discharged. The town of Tournai boasted that by pyrotechnics of this description at dawn and sunset it had ridded itself of the plague in a short time. Even a prominent physician like Sorbait supported this idea, and for him the vitiation of the air was proved not only by the astral conjunctions, but by the departure of the birds, by the dying of canaries and cats as well as by the large numbers of toads. Many people had little birds flying about in their rooms so that they might absorb the poison and keep the air in motion. It was also believed that spiders, particularly the larger and speckled species, absorbed all poison in the houses, thus preserving the inhabitants from infection. " On which account they were carefully preserved as conscientious purifiers of the air and permitted to spin their webs everywhere." The same faculties of absorption were attributed to toads and lizards, as was believed by Helmont; "if dried, they are brought into contact with the body, as is also the case with diamonds, almandine, sapphire and topas, and particularly with jasper engraved with a scorpion." Dishes with new milk were frequently placed in the rooms and were supposed to absorb the poisonous air. Some experimented with warm or new baked bread, that was stuck up on a stick in the air. A piece of warm bread was laid on the mouth of the dying to catch the poison which was supposed to develop most virulently at the moment of expiration. Large flocks of oxen and cows were driven through many towns, that by their breath they might improve the air. Cardanus attributes the same property to the breath of horses and recommends living in a stable. In the Balkans and in many places in Germany it was believed that the air could be changed by means of stinks. Leather, boot soles, buck's horn were used for fumigating. In the Crimea numbers of dead dogs were thrown in the streets. The maddest of all was that stinking billy-goats were constantly kept in living- and bed-rooms. The Chief Chancellor of Hungary is said to have had a large billy-goat in his room. Gruling reports that in a butcher's house where a goat was kept no one died. Rivius, on the other hand, in his book on the plague at Leipzig, states that houses with stinking billy-goats were infected. The first to sing the praises of the billy, he says, stank himself like a rutting buck, and was called Pamphilus or Loveall, but he only loved girls who smelt like goats.

According to the observations of some authors, tanners and people engaged in cleaning out latrines as well as servants at inns remained immune from the scourge. The tanners doubt-less owed their immunity to the tannin contained in the bark. Rommel relates that it was actually recommended to stand early in the morning on an empty stomach above a latrine and inhale the stench. "But I cannot conceive what benefit can be derived from this, particularly by sensitive people, who can hardly bear it if the air in the room is vitiated by someone. How could such a stench prove beneficial to them which is so horrible and is due to the excrements of all kinds of persons, healthy and sick, and to all kinds of rubbish and filth which have been thrown in? Quite on the contrary I believe that such poisonous stinks are rather the cause of more easy infection, although a certain medical man maintains the contrary, and believes that a certain town in Holland owes its immunity from the plague, which was raging quite close to it, solely to its piggish filth; but I think this is not the reason and other causes must exist to which this should be attributed. Besides, how can that be beneficial in times of plague which is not good at other times, but disgusting, and most repulsive, so that one covers one's mouth and nose; unless indeed any person should have a strange liking and secret affinity for such-like filth, so that his heart would be more easily comforted by dirt and filth than by the scent of musk and amber and other refreshing things—as I myself once made the acquaintance of such a filth-lover who preferred the smell of pigs' dung to anything else, and could thoroughly enjoy it. But here the saying is applicable: 'What does a cow care for mace?'

Such filthmongers may be left to enjoy their stinks and may, if they wish for nothing better, absorb them to their full." But these filth therapeutists had the support of an eminent authority—Paracelsus, who taught that in times of plague all excrements, but particularly human excrements, were healthy.

Diderich reports of a fire philosopher who recommended " bottled wind," but adds that he did not state how the bottling was to be done. A monk recommended goat urine ; Abraham Hossmann writes : " A wash with urine does more than any other preventive, more particularly when in addition the urine was drunk." He also relates that two lovers at Liegnitz during the plague determined to stay together till death. Every day they made themselves a bath of their own urine and by this means were preserved from the greatest danger.

Rommel writes : " Some praise most highly that a man should drink his own urine of a morning, as this counteracts constipation of the liver, the spleen, etc., prevents putrefection in the stomach and elsewhere ; and this may be admitted, and is certainly of greater value, than to absorb the stinks of privy places, particularly if the person is of a healthy constitution."

An " experienced plague physician " expresses as his opinion, " that at one place those who have to bury plague dead preserved themselves by means of their own urine by mixing it with a little cuckoldwort, wormwood, and ironwort, after which it is strained through a cloth and a drink prepared from it." This same much-travelled imperial physician mentions, further, that in the hospital or plague house of Paris the barbers and such persons who tend the sick, and take off and clean their plasters and dirty dressings, among other preventives use their own urine, but in the following manner : " They take their own urine, put it in a glazed pot and boil it until it is evaporated to a salt ; after this they take a good knife-point full of this salt on a piece of bread which has been dipped in sweet oil and eat it early of a morning on an empty stomach, drink a good draught of herb wine, and when in contact with their patients they chew a bit of plaguewort. By those much is said in praise of *Sal Urinæ*, and it is at the discretion of any man to do the same." It was particularly known of the old corpse-washer of Leipzig, who had closed the eyes of more than a thousand plague patients, that " it was only by means of his urine that he preserved himself, and that every morning he drank a handful of it in the name of the Father, the Son, and the Holy Ghost." But not only by means of urine, but also by menstrual blood, the plague was said to be successfully overcome.

" The gentle reader," Guarinonius writes on one occasion, " must not be too sensitive, as it is not always possible to treat of beautiful, clean things, as even a prince and potentate on a long journey must occasionally pass through a puddle when this is decreed by the roughness and unevenness of the road."

Extraordinarily popular were the various amulets and heart-bags which were sold and prescribed mainly by quacks, old women, and begging friars, but also by physicians. Guy de Chauliac, who no longer believed in the sorcery and magic which, particularly later on in the sixteenth and seventeenth centuries, claimed so many victims in Europe, yet recommended to follow the advice of Hermes, and in times when the sun was in the sign of the Lion and the moon did not turn towards Saturn to don a belt of lion-skin, which in pure gold and as clearly cut as possible should bear the image of a lion. Cardanus, on whom precious stones had such a magic effect that an emerald which he placed on his tongue and held in his mouth appeased the violent grief which he felt at the death of his son, praises the hyacinth-stone " because it bears such similitude to the human spirit, gives joy and comfort and, worn near the heart, preserves from plague." Particularly pregnant women should wear all kinds of precious stones on neck and hands, and as often as possible touch the left breast with them. In their drinking-cups they should at all times have " real unicorn," for this revives the heart and corporeal spirits and preserves from pestilential infection. If they fall ill, they should drink red wine in which a new steel has been cooled several times; should hold bloodstones in their hands and frequently pass them from one hand to the other. Should also put ground red coral in their wine. A certain bone from the head of a toad attached to the breast is said to protect against every infection. Paracelsus writes " that against timid imagination or anxiety, which kills the greater part of

humanity, the venomous tongues of snakes attached to the
body are very good." When Henry II of France was
besieging Metz and the plague broke out in his army, the
leaders as well as the sick attendants are said to have protected themselves by wearing hollowed-out hazel-nuts filled
with " live mercury " round their necks. Others recommended arsenic or tragacanth made into a paste and wound
round with silk, to be worn on the heart. Thus the Sibylla
made a great mystery of nine letters which are said to have
been the word " Arsenicum." Celebrated Italian physicians,
based on the principle that one poison counteracts another,
are said to have attached great value to arsenic, and Pope
Hadrian VI is said to have been preserved by an arsenic
amulet that he wore above his heart. Daniel Defoe relates
how in London during the Great Plague such amulets were
worn by nearly everyone, particularly also spells, signs from
the zodias, papers fastened with so and so many knots on
which certain words or figures were inscribed, among which
the mysterious triangle " Abracadabra " was specially
prominent :

```
ABRACADABRA
ABRACADABR
ABRACADAB
ABRACADA
ABRACAD
ABRACA
ABRAC
ABRA
ABR
AB
A
```

In conjunction with fervent prayers and true repentance
the anagram or transmutation of the letters " *Pestilentia lenit
Pietas* " worn as an amulet was said to be very efficacious. To
this class of plague amulets belong the plague pennies which
were sold particularly in Poland by the mendicant friars.
From Cracow it is reported that the faith in these magic
pennies was rudely shaken when the friar himself was carried
off, leaving to his smiling heirs a considerable fortune acquired
by this means. On the face of these coins the knight St.
George is depicted on horseback engaged in combat with the

dragon; the superscription was, "With God is Council and Deed." The reverse bore mystical signs with the superscription, "*Signum Rochi contra Pestem Patronus.*"

A magic prescription found on September 27, 1629, at Herzogenbusch on the evacuation of the Spanish runs :

"The Roman Emperor sent to our Holy Father, the Pope, for advice against the plague. The Pope answered thus : These holy names should be worn against it :

"Jesus, Mary, Anna, Micheal, Bernardus, Niclajus, Sebastianus, Christofolus, Martinus, Silvester, Rochus, Fredergus, and Gutrudus.

"And there should be read fifteen paternosters and five Ave Marias and seventeen rosaries; in the space of nine days this should be done once.

"He who does this shall not die of the plague, for it has been tried in many towns in which the plague prevailed, and by the hand of God it has been staid in the selfsame hour.

"This is the Will of God and of our Beloved Lady, and of his blessed five wounds which neither swelled nor festered ; thus do I hope that this plague will not swell.

"In the name of the Father ✠, of the Son ✠, and of the Holy Ghost ✠.

Good St. Adrian stabbed his hand
He spoke and blessed against the plague this brand.

"In the name of the Father ✠, of the Son ✠, and of the Holy Ghost ✠. Amen.

Jesus Christus, natus est   I.
Jesus Christus crucifixus est   II.
Jesus Christus sepultus est   III.
✠ Amen.

"This ye must inscribe on a scroll of paper and daily eat one.

✠ Christus ✠ natus ✠
✠ Christus ✠ passus ✠
✠ Christus ✠ a mortuis resurrexit ✠

"This ye must inscribe on a paper folded seven times to the number of five times, and every day on empty stomach eat one, saying the while five paternosters and five Ave Marias."

During the Plague of Naples in 1657 the philosopher and physician Morexanus wore upon his breast as amulet a Latin letter of the Mother of God. The letter ran: "The Virgin Mary, Joachim's daughter, the humble handmaiden of God, the mother of Christ Jesus, crucified, of the race of Judah and the family of David, sends greetings to all inhabitants of Messina, and sends to them the blessing of God, the Father Almighty. Ye have all, as is well known, with great confidence sent unto me ambassadors and messengers with a public letter. Ye confess that my son was born of God, was himself God and man, and after his resurrection ascended into heaven. Ye are acquainted with the way of truth by the preaching of the selected apostle Paul. Therefore do I bless you and the citizens, and will for ever be your guard and protection. In the year of my son 1642, Thursday, the 27th day of June, dated at Jerusalem. The Virgin Mary, who vouches for the above handwriting." This letter cropped up again during the plague at Messina in 1743 and is said to have diffused a sweet perfume over a radius of ten miles.

Diderich relates how the honest people of Leipzig tore off all the amulet rubbish from their necks and laid aside the golden rings and chains before their deaths, and how Pater du Bruyn, a learned Jesuit, did away with three or four boxes containing images, sacred relics, and consecrated scrolls and the like in great disgust before his death, saying: " Oh, ye vain supports on which I have relied ! " " This wretchedness," Diderich continues, " will come to an end when the people become as knowing as sheep, which do not entrust their lives to a hungry wolf."

A good many may have fared like the Erfurt carpenter who, after having experienced indifferent luck, in a fit of impatience tore open the scroll contained in his amulet and read the words :

> To him who bears this note along
> A joyful hour ne'er belong,
> Who in these words with trust confides
> Within his skin a great fool hides.

The great Florentine satirist Poggio relates in his "*Facetiæ*," under the title "Plague Talisman," the following story: "When recently staying at Tivoli on a visit to my children, whom I had sent there from Rome, on account of the plague, I heard a curious story which I must insert in my 'Tales and Stories.' A few days before a monk, one of those who wander about in the country and preach in the neighbouring villages to the peasants, had promised them an amulet, as they are called; if they wore it round their necks they could never die of the plague. The peasants, a stupid lot, were tempted by it, bought the amulets and wore them attached by a new string round their necks. The monk had said that no one was to open the amulet before fourteen days had elapsed, otherwise it would lose its power. He raked in a great quantity of money and decamped.

"Later on the amulets were read—curiosity is the besetting vice of mankind—and there stood written in the vulgar tongue:

Donna, sè fili, e cadeti lo fuso.
Quando te fletti, tien lo culo chiuso.

If spinning your spindle should fall to the ground
In bending be careful and don't make a sound.

That far surpasses all that physicians could prescribe."

As a very important and very rational means of preservation it was considered that in times of plague the bowels should be kept particularly open; "for during constipation the body is subject to infection by illness, and particularly in times of plague it is very dangerous for a man to be swollen up and filled with moisture."

A curious preventive measure was the blistering of the thighs by means of Spanish flies, burning herbs, or surgical operation. The wounds were kept open artificially during the whole duration of the plague, and fresh butter or lard was rubbed into them. Thomas Plater relates of a member of some order who pierced the testicles of all his brethren in the monastery, and also operated on many other people, instead of using a seton he used a white hellebore and thus preserved them from the plague.

All remedies with which the patients were treated aimed mainly at a restriction of putrefying tendencies and a stimulation of the heart. To some extent they were quite good, but for the most part they recall the words of Goethe's " Faust " :

> Here was the medicine, the patients died,
> And no one asked : Who then was healed ?
> And thus with devilish confections
> We raged within these mountains and these dales
> Much worse than e'er the plague.

As in all mediæval therapeutics, which bear the mark of Arabian influence, complicated and curious formulæ play a great part. The more filthy and disgusting the substances prescribed the greater the power of healing appeared to be. The physicians of Perugia attributed the deadliness of the plague to small worms, which they maintained they had found in particularly large numbers in the vicinity of the heart. Against these worms theriaca as well as the juice of scabiosa and hyssop was prescribed. Chrysopolitanos prescribes as a remedy of great virtue strong capon essence : " Take a good fat capon or a good fowl, cut up into small pieces, grind the bones thoroughly, then place it in a glass retort to distil, and if it be desired to make the essence still stronger, pearls, ducats, red corals, or precious stones may be added, and this essence should be frequently administered to the patient. A heart-warmer may be made in the following manner :

Take :
> Flesh coloured wild roses
> Borage blossoms
> Ox tongue blossoms
> Rosemary blossoms
> Balm mint blossoms or the herb, 2 drachms of each
> Camphor, 2½ drachms
> Best balm, 1 scruple
> Hyacinth powder
> Prepared emerald
> Prepared garnet, ½ scruple
> Red and white ground sandal-wood
> Red coral, 1 drachm
> Saffron, 2 drachms
> Ground silver
> Ground gold leaves, 2 of each.

With all these things a heart-warmer is made in the form of a little silk bag. Then take a warm brick, sprinkle it with rose-

water, and lay the bag on the brick, and when it has become
heated place on the heart of the patient."

The bezoar stone was held in high esteem. The celebrated
English physician Boyle was, however, of opinion " that a
stone that had grown in a human being was of much greater
avail in times of plague." The plague elixir of Tycho de
Brahe was frequently applied, and was supposed to produce a
beneficial turn in the disease by inducing the patient to sweat.
The main drug against the plague, and one which was used in
all countries without exception, was theriaca of snakes.

In the first instance, the supposed obvious healing properties of this remedy may be attributed to religious considerations. " Not only did the serpent bring down upon us great
and eternal tribulation by the fall of our first ancestors, but
there is also a lasting enmity between man and the serpent,
because its bite is injurious to us and its sting is mortal. But,
however injurious it may be to us, we may yet expect some
good from it ; for, not to mention that if with true eyes of
faith we gaze on the serpent raised on Mount Golgotha we are
delivered from all poison in our souls and from the sting of
conscience, and may become capable of the grace of God and
eternal bliss, the snake is of great importance and use in
medicine, as it is found to be efficient against diseases,
especially against poison."

The most remarkable pharmacopœic production of the
seventeenth century, " *La Thériaque Française*," by Pierre
Maginet, an apothecary of Salins, 1623, sings the praise of all
the virtues and qualities of this renowned remedy and gives a
lucid description of its preparation :

> The master well skilled in the theriac art,
> The female alone for his work sets apart,
> When in spring from its deeply hid lair it escapes
> On the fresh greening meadows its coils it now shakes.
> No young must she bear in her body as yet,
> And her eyes must be red as the sun at its set,
> Her neck must be slender and her tail of such shape
> That, though moderate of length, like a lance it should tape.
> I state it quite clearly, a head broad and smooth,
> For by this the distinction 'twixt viper and serpent is couth.

And now to prepare without further delay
On the back of the beast with a rod he must lay
To excite it to anger, that the poison may swell
And flood with its inrush throat and fangs well.

Through the teaching of Paracelsus it became usual to lay dried toad on the plague boils. " For the other plague which has collected and formed a centre," he writes, " toads should be taken which have been dried thoroughly in the air or the sun and they should be laid on the boil, then the toad will swell and draw the poison of the plague through the skin to itself, and when it is full it should be thrown away and a new one applied ; no one should feel disgust at the use of such physic. For thus God has ordered it that the poison of the plague should be drawn out by dried toads, for then one evil thing serves to extract another. But if toads are not to be procured, I have seen that a cock was taken and its posterior plucked, and thus bare and alive applied, and that the cock died and collected all the poison in itself. Living sparrows are said to have the same effect."

If during the plague delirium and inflammation of the brain ensue, " a young pigeon should be taken and torn asunder and, still warm, applied to the head, in the same manner a puppy dog of one month old may be used. Of extraordinary interest are reports from Poland, where, at Warsaw, when nothing could be found to stay the plague, the boils of the dead were cut out, dried, powdered, and given to the sick, as is maintained with success. Johann Christian Kundmann relates that this remedy " is particularly efficacious as a preservative against the plague so as to enable intercourse with those infected and the nursing of them." Many, particularly among the poor, were so courageous that they swallowed the pus from the mature boils in spoonfuls. Wilhelm Sahm, in his history of the plague in East Prussia, relates the same from the district of Labiau, where the peelings of plague boils were given to those who remained healthy in their food and drink. That plague pus in itself is not necessarily infectious is corroborated by various authors on the plague. The best-known case is that of the celebrated theologician Justus Jonas, who as a little boy ate the baked onion which had been lying on his father's boil and had then been forgotten at the bedside, and which did him no harm at all. The most positive treatment during the plague was undoubtedly the surgical operation as executed by Guy de Chauliac and, following his example, by all other physicians. The boils were cut open and burnt out with hot irons—an operation which, as Hecker affirms, was at all times successful and saved innumerable people.

Finally, a few German proverbs may serve to show how sceptical the people were in regard to medical treatment of the plague, which they designated by such names as " Hans Mors the Longlegs," " Robber Quick," and " Hasty Booter."

" In times of plague smallpox is vague."

" The plague has no fear of the apothecary."

" If the plague begs for a penny, give it two and let it go."

" If once the plague is in the house it stays there long."

" The plague attacks those first who are most afraid."

" The plague lasted seven years, but no one died before his time."

" The best means against the plague is a pair of new boots used till they break."

> The plague at first on those does fall
> Whose food and drink is rich withal.

APPENDIX

THE UNIVERSAL PRESCRIPTION OF ABRAHAM A SANTA-CLARA

All-knowing, all-ordering, and most wise God has pre-scribed, even for the animals deprived of reason, certain herbs and roots of the earth to which in sickness and frailties of the body they have recourse. Stags, when they feel ill, cure them-selves with the herb dictam ; the bear when sick heals himself with ivy ; the lizard when ill with the leaves of the wild lettuce ; the cat when its eyes fail uses the herb neptin ; the fowls and turtle-doves if not in good health are cured with the herb called "day and night," in latin *Parietaria* ; the swallows are cured by herbs and the snake cures itself with fennel.

Even the dirty snail cures itself with the herb cunila or thyme. There is no animal, however small or insignificant, for whom God has not prescribed some medicine among the herbs of the fields and the roots of the earth; and should there be no herb prescribed by God for man, whom he has created in His own image, against the plague? Aesculapius, Machaon, Podalirius, Serapio, Mesue, Avincenna, Apulejus—all of them men of vast experience—ascribe to the herbs and roots tormentil, bibernil, diptam, rue, valerian, angelica, borage, etc., so strong an effect that they are good and wholesome for the plague. May be; I will not dispute it. But another, a better and still more wholesome herb against the plague, we, Viennese, have found; this herb is called by Plinius *Viola flammea*—some name it phlox, others use other names, but commonly it is known by the name of *Flos trinitatis* (trinity flower), and grows in all our gardens; from whence it got this name I cannot tell, but the most learned doctors never knew that this was good for the plague. Thou, O Most Wise Solomon, who knew the effect and properties of all natural things and hast treated thereof, from the cedar tree to the hyssop that breaks forth from the wall, thou didst not discern this much, that this herb is wholesome for the plague; but we, Viennese, confess it publicly, confirm it in writing and by word of mouth, affirm it irrevocably, that of all herbs and roots there has been no better remedy against the plague than *Flos trinitatis*, the flower of the trinity: to wit the most Holy Trinity—God the Father, Who created us, God the Son, Who redeemed, and God the Holy Ghost, Who hallowed us—these three most Holy Persons in one and inseparable Divinity, They have delivered us from the baneful plague, They have achieved our salvation, to Them for all eternity we owe our thanks: *Gloria Patri et Filio et Spiritui Sancto.*

CHAPTER V

ADMINISTRATIVE PRECAUTIONS

The first plague regulations—The Council of Three—Nazaretum, the island
of the plague-stricken—Moral decrees—Concubines and dice-makers—
Executed coffins—Plague bells and marked houses—Dung-hills as
burying-places—Model Marseilles—Rousseau under quarantine in the
Port of Genoa—Canonised dirt—Beneficial results of the Fire of
London.

BOCCACCIO relates that at Florence in 1348 various precautions
were taken to protect against the plague. It is also related
that during the same plague in England all communication
with Bristol, which was to lose nine-tenths of its inhabitants,
was suspended. The first plague regulation was conceived by
Visconte Bernabo at Reggio for the preservation of his life,
to which he attached great value. It is dated January 17,
1374, and states: "Everyone sick of the plague is to be brought
out of the town to the fields, there to die or recover. Those
who have nursed plague patients are to remain secluded for
ten days before having intercourse with anyone. The clergy
are to examine the sick and report to the authorities on pain
of being burnt at the stake and confiscation of their possessions.
Those who introduce the plague shall forfeit all their goods to
the State. Finally, with the exception of those set apart for
the purpose, no one shall administer to those sick of the
plague on pain of death and forfeiture of their possessions."
A prohibition to leave the town was issued, in fact more for
political than sanitary reasons, in the year 1383 by the council
of the town of Florence—"For it was to be feared that if the
most powerful were to leave the town Lord Raggle Taggle
would gain the upper hand." But this prohibition did not
retain them in the town; for the fear of the disease which had
broken out was so great that they would not stay, and the
rulers were obliged at great expense to engage special servants,

guardians and mercenaries, and introduce them into Florence to guard the town.

In Venice it is said that on March 29, 1348, for the first time a sanitary council was instituted, consisting of three noblemen. The regulations and measures drawn up by it between 1348 and 1485 have served as a model for all other European States. The island on which the Venetians isolated people and goods arriving from the Orient and confined those sick of plague was, most probably on account of the church of Santa Maria of Nazareth situated on it, called the Nazarethum, from which the word " Lazaretto " is said to be derived. The duration of isolation (quarantine) was fixed at forty days, because Christ, Moses, and so many others had remained isolated in the desert for this number of days. In 1504 the powers of the Sanitary Council were extended, and it was endowed with powers of life and death over those who came under its jurisdiction. Bills of health, or *Feden,* as they were called in Germany, were instituted in 1527 ; but they did not become general till 1665. In Germany efficacious measures of protection were adopted much later than in France and Italy. In the fourteenth century immunity was expected from *antidota spiritualia,* as the Archbishop of Prague expresses it. In the year 1463, during an outbreak of plague at Augsburg, the dead were still buried in a common grave in the centre of the town. The first German official plague regulation dates, as is related by Schoeppler in his " History of the Plague in Regensburg," from the year 1412. " Like all official publications of the time in German States and towns, it appears to be a more or less free copy of an Italian model." Considerable space is occupied in the innumerable plague regulations which were announced publicly to the sound of trumpets by moral precepts. Thus the plague regulation of the town of Rouen of the year 1507 announced that everything is to be eliminated that could cause the anger of God, such as gambling, cursing, drinking, and all excesses. In Speyer a strict prohibition had already been issued in 1347 against gambling in the churchyards, even to the extent of a halfpenny. The Council of Tournai issued an edict that all concubines were to be expelled or married, the observation of Sunday was to be strictly maintained, the manufacture and sale of dice as well as their use for gambling was to be completely suppressed. The regulation is said to have attained its purpose in regard to the first item, as numerous concubines were married. The dice factories, however, found means of adapting themselves to the tendency of the times and converted the dice into rosary beads. The plague regulation of Troyes of 1523 orders that those who have died of the plague may only be buried at night-time. The corpse-bearers, horses, and hearses must be provided with bells. Everyone who enters the town in spite of the prohibition is to be severely punished. Thus four poor women who had come from a neighbouring borough to sell old linen underclothing were condemned to be tied to a cart, driven through the town, and publicly whipped. The magistrates paid ten sous to all who took part in the whipping and forty sous to the executioner for particularly thorough work. Transgressors of the plague regulations were punished even after their death. The servant maid, Barbara Thutin, of Koenigsberg, had infected herself and her master by appropriating several articles belonging to people who had died of the plague. "As by this she had grossly contravened the strict prohibition, an execution was carried out on her after her death, she being exhumed on March 21, 1710, in the new cemetery where she had been buried, and on the 22nd hanged in her coffin on the gallows, and after a few days burnt at the foot of the gallows as an example for others." A measure to be found in nearly all plague regulations is the expulsion of drunkards, beggars, lepers, and gipsies. In many places an order was issued that all cats in plague houses should be destroyed, and that the dogs should be chained up. Cattle may not be taken over by the heirs until driven at least three times through deep water. In 1563 the inhabitants of Burgundy were ordered to refrain from using public places for the satisfaction of their physical needs, and to restrict themselves to their houses. Those who had no accommodation in their houses were to provide such immediately. The plague priests were forbidden to enter the churches and to avoid unexpected encounters with them they, as well as the surgeons, corpse-bearers, and nurses, were instructed not to walk along the houses, but in the middle of the street and to carry a bell.

Similar instructions are to be found in the sixteenth century in all countries.   Thus in Vienna corpse-bearers and nurses were marked with a white cross and provided with a peculiar pipe, so that they might warn all advancing towards them. White crosses were attached to plague houses in Thorn in 1579, and all who came from a stricken house were made to carry white wands.   In London all infected houses were marked by a red cross, " which was one foot in length and attached in the middle of the door, so that it could be distinctly seen " —right above the cross the words " Lord be merciful to us " were to be inscribed.   In Berlin in 1576, 1584, and 1598 whole streets were closed by iron chains, and municipal servants kept guard at the exits to prevent those infected or suspicious from coming out, but to provide them with necessities.

With what terrible resistance on the part of the people, not only the physicians, but also the authorities had to contend, is shown by a report of the year 1710, drawn up by two plague delegates of the Koenigsberg Sanitary Board on the conditions prevailing in the villages Neuendorf and Gallgarben : " The peasants," the report states, " resist our assistance with the utmost violence and drag the corpses of those who have died from the infection with boat-hooks from their houses to bury them in the dung-heaps beside the houses, and we have been informed that pigs have already devoured the corpses of one man and one child."   Only the threat of the authorities to punish any further resistance by burning the two places reduced the obstinate inhabitants to submission.

It was not till the beginning of the eighteenth century that a systematic scheme of protection was organised.   Marseilles, which in the year 588 experienced the first and 1720 the last of the great European epidemics of bubonic plague, by the construction of its model plague hospital and its excellent quarantine arrangements delivered France from visitations of the plague.   On the quarantine in the Port of Genoa we have a report of Jean-Jacques Rousseau from the year 1743 : " It was at the time of the plague at Messina.   The English Fleet had been in the port of Messina, and in communication with the *felucca* which conveyed Rousseau from Toulon to Genoa. That was the reason why the travellers after a long and troublesome crossing had to undergo here a quarantine of twenty-one days. They were allowed the choice of remaining on board or going to the hospital. In the latter they would, however, only find the bare walls, as there had been no time to provide the rooms with beds and utensils. All selected to remain in the *felucca*. Only Rousseau, who found the heat and restriction of space and vermin in the boat unbearable and who longed for exercise, preferred to go to the hospital. He was conducted to a large two-storied bare building without windows, table, bed, or chair, in which not even a footstool offered the possibility of sitting down, or a bundle of straw of lying down. His cloak, his travelling bag, and his two trunks were brought him, and he was locked up behind two huge doors with enormous bolts, and left to wander about the rooms of the two stories, where everywhere the same emptiness and forsakenness prevailed, free to make his own arrangements like a new Robinson Crusoe. His meals were brought him and placed on the staircase by a prison warder, accompanied by two gendarmes with guns and fixed bayonets, and announced by ringing a bell. The influence of the French Minister, to whom he managed to have conveyed a letter soaked in vinegar and half burnt, was successful in having his imprisonment reduced by a week " (" Confessions," ii. 7). The most striking case of the infringement of quarantine regulations is supplied by Bonaparte on his return from Egypt on October 9, 1798. What a difference it would have made to Europe if Sieyès had succeeded with his motion to have the great infringer of the law shot.

Of the greatest importance for the suppression of the plague, which by modern scientists is reckoned among diseases due to dirt, was the increase in cleanliness and civilisation throughout Europe. In many towns in Italy and Spain in the fourteenth and fifteenth centuries all filth was thrown into the yards and beside the house doors, and no thought given to the construction of cesspools or middens. In 1610 Guarinonius complains that in many houses in Germany there are still no privies. It is well known that in the mediæval ages people did not wash every day, and that they wore their clothes till they fell off as rags. Saint Agnes was canonised because she refused to bathe. What the historian David Hume writes in 1757 on the consequences of the Great Fire of London in 1666 is of great interest. " After the Great Fire the town was very rapidly reconstructed, and attention was paid to making the streets broader and more regular than before. Great as this calamity was, yet greater advantages were derived from it, for after the fire London was much more healthy. The plague which generally broke out with great vehemence twice or thrice a century, and in fact every time appeared first in the most filthy corner of the town, has never been heard of since this great misfortune."

Experience gained during the various epidemics of plague contributed everywhere essentially to the consideration of hygienic aspects in the construction of towns and dwellings. But the most important factor in the restriction of the plague was the definite expulsion of the Turks from Europe.

A plague cordon was erected against the Balkan peninsula and quarantine institutions established along the coasts of the Adriatic and Mediterranean. In the nineteenth century the plague only appeared in Greece (1827), at Odessa (1839), in Syria, Egypt, and Turkey (1835). Since 1841 it has not broken out in these countries, thanks to the sanitary and plague police introduced into Turkey.

CHAPTER VI

ATTITUDE OF THE CHURCH

The plague as Divine punishment—Theatre, pointed shoes, and luxurious clothes arouse the wrath of God—Royal misalliances as cause of plague—Monastic quarrels—Excommunication of comets, mice, and insects—A French mouse trial—Self-sacrifice and pious fraternities—Saint Rochus—Venetian adventurers—Superstitious views—Plague prayers—The emerald of Clement IV—Origin of the Dance of Death—The miracle of the monastery at Milan—Bishop Henri de Castel Moron, the Saviour of Marseilles—The Church inherits immense wealth—Martin Luther—Justifiable resentment of the lower classes—Religious stoicism in the maritime towns—Hymns and spiritual verse.

Appendix : The plague in the monastery of St. Gall, A.D. 1629.

UNTIL the beginning of the seventeenth century the opinion was prevalent that God inflicted the plague upon man as a punishment for his sins " because the ways of humanity were inhuman, and we men did not love our neighbours, but that all our doings turned towards luxuriant living." This opinion found particular support in the Church, and was maintained even in the eighteenth century when the plague made its last appearance at Marseilles in 1720. During the Black Death the whole of Europe was persuaded that the end of the world was approaching. The plague was the apocalyptic rider on the pale horse, and all signs which were said to precede the last day were recognised which had been prophesied by Christ, the prophets, and the apostles.

An author gives a humorous turn to the punitive theory in 1640 : " That we may know this and how it all comes to pass I will relate you a parable. An innkeeper has in his house undesirable guests and would fain be rid of them, but does not know how to set about it decently; he tries to drive them out by stench and foul odours—he could find no other means; he takes leather, horns, hoofs, claws, woollen cloth, feathers, asafœtida, and evil-smelling things, and makes a heap of them and sets it alight. The smoke rises and smells horrible, the guests bid him farewell, etc. Thus also God behaves in Nature when he wishes to punish sinful men ; he makes a pungent smell—that is, the poisoned air. What ingredients does he take ? These are first his poisonous stars, the baneful aspects and planets, etc. God has quick postal messengers. He can transmit his messages with speed, for thus you have deserved it. He is omnipotent ; for a small draught proved so strong, as is reported by the historians, in Seleucia when the men-at-arms of Emperor Antonius wished to break open a shrine in the church of Apolonis, believing that they would find money in it, but they only found a whirlwind, a stench, which filled all Greece with pestilence and subsequently passed to Rome and all Europe. How quickly God can prepare such a whirlwind and make his angels blow it forth into all countries, can be read in the Apocalypse in all parts."

According to Luther it is the devil whom God uses as executioner in such cases : " Thus he punishes us by the Devil, who is always our enemy, and, if God did not prevent him, would destroy us all in a moment. Like a dog he is fastened with a chain, so that he may do us no harm unless we wantonly go to him of our own accord, till God on account of our sins releases him from his chain so that he may run up and down and bite whomsoever he may encounter." The sins on account of which God is said to have inflicted the plague on man would appear to us to-day in some respects very trivial. Thus the Spanish clergy attribute the outbreak of the plague to the opera, the English bishops in the year 1563 to the theatre. Particularly the long-pointed shoes which had just come into fashion at the time of the Black Death were supposed to have caused special annoyance to God. The heavily visited inhabitants of Frammerbach in the Spessart in 1607 still believed that they could appease God by a vow that all women on Sundays and holidays should only wear black blouses and black skirts, and the men only grey clothes. In France an epidemic of plague was explained by the three sons of King Philip " having married in prohibited degrees of relationship, on which account they had no luck, for all their three wives proved faithless to them. Sins of this kind are frequently the cause why God punishes a whole country."

In Poland in the year 1572 a great epidemic of plague broke out because a sorceress had been buried in the church at Lemberg. The corpse was exhumed; " then it was found that she had a piece of her dress in her mouth, as if seized by sudden hunger ; her head was severed with a spade and the corpse covered with earth, whereupon the plague abated." More than once Catholics and Protestants mutually and simultaneously attributed the blame for God's anger to one another. Thus, when in 1529 the English sweating disease passed into Germany the Romanists raised their voices and said " that a new religion must necessarily be followed by a new torment of villains." In the year 1552 the plague was caused in the opinion of the Protestants " by the divergence of Church doctrine in many supreme articles, particularly such bearing on the Holy Sacraments and the blood of our dear Lord Jesus Christ." At the time of the Renaissance pride, defiance, and haughtiness particularly aroused the anger of God. Saint Carlo Borromeo, the hero of the Milan plague of the year 1526, reproached his beloved town in touching words with its sins : " O town of Milan, thy greatness and sublimity raised thee to the skies, thy riches extended to the borders of the earth. Men, animals, birds, all lived and increased on thy abundance. From all kinds of places and remote corners people of less degree flocked to thee to gain their living under thy shadow in the sweat of their brows. There came to thee the nobles and lords to dwell in thy mansions, and enjoy thy advantages and settle in thy territory. And now, behold ! in the space of a moment thy haughtiness has been humbled to scorn and defiance, and in the eyes of the world thou hast become suddenly an object of derision. Thou art restricted to thy own town walls; thy enterprise and trade and superabundance have been suppressed within thyself. No one comes to take up his dwelling in thy midst or to subsist on thy fruits, to make provision of thy wares, to clothe themselves in thy precious cloths, thy gold and silver brocade, to repose on thy couches, to enjoy thy pleasures and advantages, much less to adorn themselves with the inventions of thy new vanity, nor to acquire from thee models of new magnificence. Away from thee fled high and low, the noble like the common herd deserted thee, and he who did not flee from thee, he fled either from the baneful disease or from doubtful touch and intercourse to the anxieties of the plague refuge or outside the town, thinking it great luck and mercy if he procured sufficient straw to cover himself, as for miles

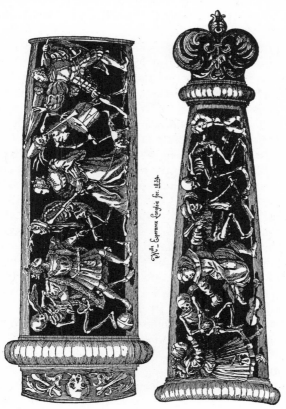

TWO DAGGER SHEATHS.
After Hans Holbein.

around all straw had been used up—on account of which, O Milan, the hard ground, occasionally even water or ice, had to serve thee as a resting-place.   So that their dwelling to a great extent was under the open sky, under the dew, the rain, the winds, outside in the midst of the fields and in places where the cattle and other beasts feed, and a strong guard of soldiers was set over thee lest thou shouldst escape from thy tribulations. Thy streets and lanes, thy houses, the squares, the churches, the shops, all stand forsaken and closed ; thou sad and miserable town of Milan, thou who didst require for thy necessary subsistence to be provided by the neighbouring towns and markets, yea even by the poor villages. Thou, Milan, wert, so to say, beside thyself, maddened by fearful terror, deprived of all thy senses. Thus the just anger of God has humbled all thy pride and haughtiness."

Boccaccio reports that processions instituted by the Church and all humble supplications to God were of no avail. Was it the corruption of the Church itself that had so aroused the wrath of God ? A witness of the Black Death at Siena, Donato Dineri, gives in a few lines a graphic description of the corruption which prevailed among the clergy, particularly among the monks. " The friars of the Order of St. Augustine at St. Antonio stabbed their provincial head. A young lay brother from Camporeggi slew another brother of the monastery, the son of Carlo Montamini ; yea, at Assisi the Minor Friars fought with knives so that fourteen of them were killed, and the Friars della Rocca di Siena did away with six of their companions. In Certosa also unrest broke out, so that the head of the Order was obliged to transfer many monks to other monasteries. Things had come to such a pass that all monks lived in disunity and strife. In Siena there was no truth or honesty to be found among men, even the honesty of the nobility was not to be relied on. Thus the whole world was shrouded in darkness. *Cosi il mondo è una tenebra.*"

The Church on various occasions pronounced against the fatalistic opinion that certain conjunctions of the stars were the cause of the plague. In astrology she perceived remnants of paganism, and Cecco d'Ascoli, who cast the nativity of Christ and from it deduced His death on the Cross, was in 1327 condemned to be burnt at the stake. In spite of this most of the popes publicly consulted the stars, and of Paul III we know that he never held a consistorium without having previously had the hour determined by astrologers. On the other hand, a sinister significance was attributed to comets by the Church. Thus the Pope excommunicated the comet which appeared in 1532, and a ban was placed on the grubs, caterpillars, locusts, rats, mice, and even cockchafers as precursors of the plague in 1478 by the Bishop of Berne, 1516 by the Bishop of Troyes, and 1541 by the Bishop of Lausanne. A particularly remarkable action was taken against mice in France in 1540. The circumstances of this legal farce are : " In certain districts of France the mice had completely devoured the corn in the fields and done immense damage. The rural population were greatly incensed, but did not know how to wreak their vengeance on the vermin. At last it occurred to them that they could do no better than to lodge a complaint against the mice with the bishop, requesting him to pronounce a ban on them, then they would be rid of them once and for all. Immediately they drew up and submitted their complaint, requesting the grant of the needed official protection. The bishop summoned a consistorium and discussed this difficult case with the clergy. The opinion of all was that the request of the poor people must be granted. But in order to condemn no one without having heard his defence, they decided that it was necessary to summon the mice three times; this was then done. When, then, the mice did not put in an appearance the bishop still refrained from pronouncing the ban, and maintained that before this could be done a counsel must be appointed for the accused who could plead for the absentees. The counsel did his best, and pointed out to the judges that the mice had not been served with summons in the legal manner, and that therefore they could not be expected to appear, and he attained that much that the mice were once more summoned from all pulpits for a certain day. Although the mice remained irresponsive and did not appear, their counsel still set forth how it was impossible for the mice to arrange an appearance in so short a time, and pleaded for an extension. In addition they had not been assured of safe-conduct, and had therefore not been able to come. Everywhere in villages, towns, and on the roads the cats cruelly waylaid them. He therefore begged to delay judgment. The case was adjourned *sine die*."

Concerning the behaviour of the priests during the great plague of 1348 very various reports have been preserved. In Italy the clergy were seized by the general terror of death, and everywhere thousands perished without the comfort of the Holy Sacraments. Thus Pompejo Pellini relates in his history of Perugia that no friar or priest was to be found to hear confession and to converse with the sick, and no one to accompany them to the grave. In France, and particularly in Germany, the priests were much more devoted. In order to avoid infection, however, the host was offered at the end of a pole or small staff with a ferule, or in a long-handled spoon. It was not permitted to offer it if the tongue of the dying man was dry or his throat was swollen, or in cases of constant coughing, hiccoughing, and vomiting. The extreme unction was not to be given to the infected. If this was done, however, cottonwool was dipped into the consecrated oil, and this was fastened to a rod or staff and inserted through a hole in the door (the plague hole), and the face of the patient touched with it if it could be reached.

An example of striking fearlessness and priestly devotion to duty is registered by St. Charles in his book "*Memoriale al suo diletto populo*" (Recollections of His Beloved People) : "One night a man infected by the plague had been laid together with the corpses of others who had died of the disease and driven to the cemetery near the plague hospital of St. George and thrown upon a heap of corpses there, according to the custom, to wait till the following morning, and then to be blessed with the rest and buried in the earth. When next morning the priest of the plague hospital of St. George was passing with the Holy Sacrament of the altar on his way to some dying plague patients, and the miserable man crawling about among the corpses caught sight of him, he raised himself as far as he could upon his knees amongst the corpses in the ardent desire, if any way possible, to receive the celestial food. He applied to the priest and addressed him in a most beseeching and touching voice, saying, ' O father, for the sake of God give me the Most Holy Sacrament.' Beyond these words, which were sufficient to prove how ardently he desired to comfort his soul with the angelic food, he was, on account of his weakness, incapable of saying anything. The love and devotion of the priest was so great that without hesitation he approached him to comfort him and grant him his request. And when he now with great devotion and respect had received the most holy and consecrated bread he lay down in the same place among the dead and expired immediately."

Of Tauler it is also related that he distinguished himself by great intrepidity. It is said that at Strasburg at the time of a great plague epidemic in the years 1349 and 1350 he administered the Sacrament to all who desired it. Extraordinarily good work was done by the various pious fraternities which were founded for tending the sick and burying the dead. In the year 1180 the fraternity of St. Eligius, one of

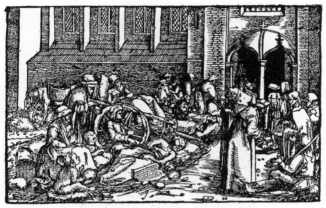

PLAGUE SICK IN FRONT OF CHURCH.
Woodcut by H. Weiditz.

the apostles of Flanders, was founded. It flourished particularly in Normandy. It is related that the Brothers of the Order carried plague corpses in their arms to burial. Four hundred of them remained free from infection. "When they had completed this task they returned unharmed to their families." Fearless and indefatigable were also the Poor Friars, whose Order was founded by a certain Tobias on the middle course of the Rhine in the middle of the fourteenth century. In a bull of Eugene IV (1431) they are described by the name of Cellites—which has now become usual, Cella being equivalent for grave—or as Burying Friars. In the year 1348 Bernhard Tolomail, the founder of the congregation of the Most Holy Virgin of Monte Olievto, met with death while nursing the

sick of the plague. In the same manner Gerhard Groote,
founder of the community called Brethren of the Common
Life or Friar Lords, died of the plague on August 20, 1384,
a victim of his active love of humanity. Groote was one of
the favourite disciples of J. van Rueysbruek. On June 21,
1591, Aloysius of Gonzaga succumbed to the infection in
Rome after having tended and comforted innumerable sufferers.
He was canonised by the Church. In Vienna the fraternity
of St. Sebastian was founded to combat the plague. They

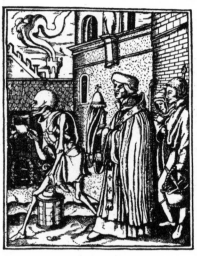

THE PARISH PRIEST.
Woodcut by Holbein the Younger.

preserved in the Scottish Church among their relics one of the
original arrows which were drawn from the corpse of the
martyr St. Sebastian. On this saint's day silver arrows,
after having been touched by the original arrow, were blessed
by the priest and distributed among the congregation; wine
which had previously passed through the skull of the martyr
at Eversberg was also dispensed through a hollow arrow, and
a particle of the bone of the arm was offered to be kissed. All
this as a preservative against infection.

During the plague at Marseilles the Capucins and Jesuits
distinguished themselves; they hastened from all quarters of

the world to place themselves at the service of those attacked by the plague. At that time members of these Orders were to be seen in the streets of Marseilles who had hardly recovered from the disease, and still covered with plague boils dragged themselves along on their sticks to hear the confessions of the dying.

A particularly interesting feature of the Middle Ages are the ecclesiastic fraternities of fools which were founded to combat the fear of death—for instance, " The Company of the Fool " of Aarau under the patronage of the plague saint St. Sebastian and the Virgin Mary. Unfortunately no details concerning them have been preserved, and we only know that on the outbreak of great epidemics they cheered the hearts of the people by public masquerades and processions.

Prayers and vows were the two main spiritual means by which the Church endeavoured to combat the plague. As in ancient times, on the outbreak of epidemics statues and altars were raised to the gods, now churches, and costly pillars were erected in the honour of the Holy Trinity, the Divine Virgin Mary, and various saints; at Vienna to the Holy Trinity, at Venice to the Divine Virgin, the liberator, at Milan to St. Sebastian, at Naples to the Divine martyr Blasius, at Madrid and innumerable other towns to St. Rochus ; in Sicily to St. Rosalie. Since the seventh century St. Sebastian was regarded as the patron saint of the plague, when during a great outbreak in Rome someone had a revelation that the plague would not yield till in the church of St. Peter an altar was erected in honour of St. Sebastian. So soon as this was done the plague ceased. That supplication to St. Sebastian was followed by a subsidence of the plague is frequently confirmed in later times.

The real plague saint of the mediæval ages is St. Rochus, one of the most amiable figures of this period. Titian, Tintoretto, Rubens, Guido Reni, Carracci have used his life as subjects for paintings. The festival of Rochus is one of the most popular and merry, and touched Goethe during his stay on the Rhine (August 16, 1814) so deeply that later on he presented to the Rochus chapel at Bingen a painting representing a scene from the life of the saint which had been executed from a design of his own.

Rochus was born about the middle or towards the end of the thirteenth century at Montpelier of noble and pious, but already aged, parents, John and Liberia, as the fulfilment of their prayers to the Mother of God. After having distributed the greater part of his fortune as a youth among the poor, he undertook a pilgrimage to Rome, and this at the time when the plague was raging in Italy. In the hospital of Agaspendente he had himself enrolled as an attendant, so as to practise his charity on the sufferers of the plague. Many of these he healed by signing them with the holy cross. At Rome also he occupied himself with the nursing of the sick, but was himself ultimately assailed by the plague, and fled, as he felt an impulse to violent sighing and crying and did not wish to become troublesome to his fellowmen, out of the town into the neighbouring forest, where he lay down in a solitary hut. Immediately a fresh spring of water broke out in the place, of this he drank to quench his thirst. In a country house not far from the hut of the saint there dwelt a nobleman from Piacenza whose name was Gotthard; this man perceived that his hound frequently took a piece of bread from the table and ran away. They watched it, and, lo! it made its way into the wood, where it placed the bread at Rochus's feet. The nobleman now took care of the forsaken man, and would not let him go away till he was quite restored. By his instructive intercourse with the saint Gotthard was soon so converted that he resolved to live the life of a recluse, which he carried out in the same neighbourhood. St. Rochus, having spent a considerable time at Piacenza and Cesena with the healing of plague patients and in the hut with the new recluse to confirm the latter in his new course of life, started on his journey home. Arriving at Montpelier he was recognised by no one. As at that time there was a war with Italy, he was taken for a spy and thrown into prison, where he remained for five years without making himself known, and by prayer, fasting, and vigil preparing himself for Eternity. When he felt the approach of death he asked for a priest. When the latter entered the dark prison it was suddenly lighted up by a celestial gleam, so that the priest immediately made a report to one of the town commandants. The incident was soon known throughout Montpelier, and the people hastened up in crowds to see the saint. But on opening the prison he was found to be dead. He was thirty-two years of age. It was only now that he was recognised by the red cross on his breast with which he had come into the world. On one of the walls of his prison they found a note, in which the words were written, " He who is seized by the plague and seeks refuge in Rochus will gain relief in this disease." By order of the viceroy he was solemnly entered in the main church on August 16, 1327. Some authors, however, place his death at the end of the fourteenth century and his journey to Italy in the year 1348, which would coincide better with the reports of historians on the devastations of the plague in Italy. According to Catholic belief, it has been asserted that by means of his intercession the plague was quelled in several towns, e.g. at Constance in 1414 at the time of the General Council, and at Brixen in the year 1477. It was a German youth who at Constance, when the fathers of the Council were already on the point of leaving the town, exhorted them with noble eloquence to seek refuge in St. Rochus. This exhortation was taken as a sign from heaven. With prayers and chants a grand procession was soon winding through the stricken town in honour of the saint. At its head the statue of the saint was borne, the princes of the Church followed in episcopal robes, their mitres on their heads, their crooks in their hands, led by Pope John XXIII ; in humble attitude King Sigismund, clad in royal attire, proceeded with his richly dressed suite. This procession, with all ecclesiastic splendour and secular pomp, produced a great impression on the whole population. Hardly was it over before the plague began to abate and peace once more came over the town and the council assembly. The relics of St. Rochus are at Arles and Venice. They were originally at Montpelier. Venetian adventurers, disguised as pilgrims, stole them in the year 1453 and brought them to Venice, which, owing to its commerce with the Levant, was constantly menaced by the plague. They were received by the Doge and the whole population with great rejoicings. It was resolved to build the church of San Rocco as a worthy shrine for the relics. A fraternity bearing the name of the saint was founded for the purpose of tending those sick of the plague, which later on developed into

the celebrated Scuola di San Rocco, which was adorned by
Tintoretto with scenes from the life of the saint.

The fourteen holy "friends in need," or, as they were also
called, " the fourteen martyrs," also enjoyed special veneration
as plague saints.   Further, in the mediæval ages it was a
frequent occurrence that the Monastic Orders quarrelled about
the healing properties of their saints.   Thus, for instance, the
Jesuits denied the miracles of St. Cailletan, and maintained
that the plague could only be healed by St. Sebastian or St.
Francis Xavier.   The plague prayers which have come down
to us are innumerable ; they all evoke the assistance of some
saint.   The abbess of the convent Santa Clara at Coimbra in
Portugal received during a local epidemic of plague the following
prayer to the Holy Virgin handed to her by an angel disguised
as a beggar :

> The noble star of heaven bright
> That to our Lord gave earthly light
> Has driven out and brought to naught
> The fell disease by Adam wrought.
> May this same star at present time
> Dispel from our unhappy clime
> That baneful star in power now
> That brought the plague to us below.
> Therefore, O star, so rich in love,
> Come to our aid with God above,
> To Him for our redemption pray,
> Thy fervent prayer He'll not gainsay.
> He Who thee hails His Mother still
> Will not refuse to do thy will,
> O Jesus sweet, save those from hell
> For whom Thy Mother begs so well !
> That we may gain Christ's promised wage
> O Holy Virgin God engage!

On an accompanying note there was further written : " If
the abbess and her sisters were to say and pray these lines
every day the plague would soon abate."   And this really
took place.

PRAYER TO THE HOLY MARTYR SEBASTIAN

" Holy and renowned martyr and knight of Christ, Sebastian, thou who didst prefer to forfeit the temporal favour and

honour of the tyrannical emperors Diocletian and Maxmilian than to deny Christ, and didst strengthen and comfort the Christians made captives in war, and wert therefore in the open field bound to a pillar, and so many arrows shot upon thee that thou didst resemble the porcupine ; but who by the strength of God wert soon restored to health and didst appear before the Emperor and to his face reproach him for his un-Christian conduct, upon which he had thee beaten to death with clubs and thy body thrown into a foul and loathsome pond, but which was drawn out by the Christian lady Lucinia and handed over for decent burial : I humbly beseech thee that by thy intercession to our Lord Jesus Christ we may be preserved by thy merit from plague and sudden death.   Amen ! "

PRAYER TO THE HOLY PILGRIM AND CONFESSOR ROCHUS

" O holy Rochus, thou who wert born of noble blood, and who didst distribute among the poor thy goods, and clad as pilgrim didst proceed to Rome and in Italy hast delivered multitudes of people from the plague, and hast thyself been healed of it : I supplicate thee that thou mayest obtain from God that I may find protection against the foul air empoisoned by the plague and against eternal death !   Amen."

PRAYER TO ST. ANTONY, SPECIAL PATRON AGAINST THE PLAGUE

When the sun t'wards evetide wends
All our prayer to thee ascends,
And thy praise we loudly sing,
Help in danger to us bring !
Thou who foul disease dispels,
And all illness quickly quells,
And preserves us young and old,
Thou whose love is never cold,
We are prompted evermore
In our needs thee to implore,
That for help we loudly cry
Save our souls from misery !
St. Antony, for us pray
That the hand of death God stay,
Thou who by God's strength can raise
From their graves the dead to praise,

Our need is now so great
That despair is at our gate.
We alone on thee rely,
Thy help will not let us die.
As our teacher, teach us right,
Lead, as shepherd, through the night,
Keep our hearts as virgins pure,
From all pain and danger sure.
Honour to the God of might
Honour to the Son on right,
With Holy Spirit up on high
Till to us His grace draw nigh.
Antony, to heaven we raise
Voices sounding forth thy praise.
All disease thou from us turnest
Healthful air thou to us sendest,
Elements obey thy will,
Death, from our sight hidden still,
At thy order frightened pauses,
No more terror for us causes.
Father Anton, for us pray
That Christ's promise and His mercy upon
   us descend now may.

Extraordinary comfort was provided for suffering humanity by the absolution granted by the various popes during times of plague. Clement VI promised extensive indulgences, and in the third year of his reign had a bull issued in which he granted complete absolution from all sins to all who should die on a journey to Rome, where in 1350 a Holy Year was being celebrated, and in addition ordered the angels of heaven to bear their souls straight to Paradise as he had absolved them from purgatory. The concourse to the Holy Year was immense. At Easter 1,200,000 people were counted, and again at Whitsuntide a million from all parts of Europe, who visited the churches of Rome for prayer and penance, and, chanting psalms, filled the high roads of Italy. The offerings made by the pilgrims amounted for the pope alone to seventeen million fiorini for a single year. A wit of the times remarked : "God does not desire the death of the sinner but that he should live and pay." But death also had his jubilee at Rome, and worked such havoc that of a thousand people hardly every tenth is said to have returned home. Clement VI, who at that time was at Avignon, which he had just purchased for eighty thousand gold guilders from Joan of Naples, observed at the advice of his physician in ordinary, Guy de Chauliac, who had immediately recognised the plague as an infectious disease, the greatest caution. For the whole duration of the epidemic he remained constantly in one particular apartment between two huge fires, isolated from everyone, admission to his presence being strictly prohibited. On his finger he wore as a protection against the plague an emerald which was said to have produced marvellous effects. Turned towards the south it minimised the virulence of the poison, turned to the east it reduced the possibility of infection. The plague raged to such an extent at Avignon that Clement was obliged to consecrate the Rhône so that corpses could be sunk in it. Alone in three days that followed the fourth Sunday in Lent 1,500 people died. Seven cardinals succumbed to the disease, among them the noble Giovanni Colonna, the Mæcenas of Avignon, and patron of Petrarch. At Avignon and in the County Venaissin the number of victims deplored amounted to 120,000. Among these was Petrarch's Laura, who expired in the early morning of April 6, 1348. In the year 1361 there succumbed to the plague at Avignon one hundred bishops and five cardinals. The disease also raged among the clergy during the Council of Basle in 1429. Innumerable crowds of people, including numbers of disreputable women, had flocked to the ecclesiastic assembly and brought with them death, as in 1429 the plague had already become general. He who remained at his post to which Providence had called him was a hero, like the Cardinal of Arles, who said: "I will rather hold together the assembly of the Church at the risk of my life than save my life at the risk of the assembly."

At that time four hundred people marched from Basle with crosses, banners, and priests from all the churches and monasteries to the Totenmoos in the Black Forest; five hundred sought at Einsiedeln the intercession of Our Lady; the Council to mollify her by veneration decreed that her immaculate conception should be venerated. Among the *Patres di Stabilimento* who were established on this occasion was young Æneas Sylvius, who later on became Pope Pius II. As by a miracle he recovered from a severe attack of the plague, after having been reported dead and having received the extreme

unction. Later on he furnished a detailed account of his
illness in a special book. The Assembly of Basle acquired
immortal merit alone by instituting the " Great Basle Dance
of Death." "The Dance of Death in the graveyard of the
Predicant Church was executed in oil colours about the year
1439, or two years later, by order of the Fathers of the Church
who were assembled at the Council; its cause was the plague,
which had been raging a short time before and had carried off

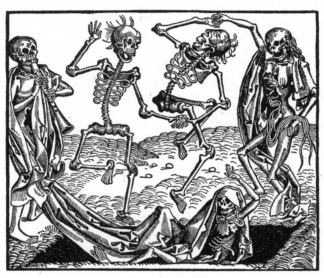

DANCE OF DEATH.
Woodcut by Mich. Wohlgemuth (?), 1493.

many important persons; it was to illustrate in the most
emphatic manner the uncertainty of human life. It would
appear that the Predicant Friars suggested as a model the
Dance of Death in the Klingenthal, with which they were
familiar." At the same time in numerous other towns and
countries Dances of Death were executed, just as poetry
again and again selected as its theme the transitory nature
of human life. The celebrated German preacher Geiler von
Kaisersperg, who in the years 1495 to 1497 preached a consecu-
tive series of sermons on death, expresses the sentiment of the
times in a simile which has become commonplace: " All

power of the world is as a pack of cards. There are various cards, some are called kings, other queens, and again others knaves. Thus, too, power is distributed on earth, one man is a king, another a mayor, and so on. Although in a pack one card is more decorative than another, and one is esteemed of more value than the other, yet they are all made of paper and cardboard stuck together. Thus, all who are endowed with power and surpass others in dignity, the lord and servant man are all fashioned of the same material, are all mortal and feeble."

Innumerable examples might be quoted to show how deeply the Church was involved in the superstitious beliefs of the mediæval ages. At Montpelier, where the plague in 1348 and 1383 was particularly virulent, the height of the walls was measured with a thread, which was then worked into a gigantic candle which was lighted on the altar of the church of Notre Dame. This peculiar ceremony was repeated in many towns, thus in Normandy at Pont Audemar in 1518. At the Council of Trent in 1546 Leonardus, the Bishop and Patriarch of Antioch, wore a bracelet, " on which was inscribed a cross with letters, that is now called the cross of St. Benedict. He informed others that it was found at Antioch in the monastery of St. Benedict, and was bequeathed by Zacharias, Bishop of Jerusalem, with interpretation, significance, and prayers, as has now (1640) been made more evident by miracles, when used devoutly and for good purpose, so that the assertions of all opponents have been silenced." Of St. Charles it is reported that he banished the plague into a marble column at Milan, as might still be seen by a boil. Before the abatement of the plague at Milan a miracle took place at the monastery on September 23, 1577, and roused the greatest sensation throughout Christendom at the time, and was reported by innumerable broadsheets, particularly in Germany. " On the 23rd of September, in the middle of the night, when many of the fathers were asleep, others still engaged in their studies or in praying in the church, whilst awaiting the hour for early Mass, suddenly the bells began to ring of their own accord. All who were awakened by them were stricken with surprise and with trembling, and hastened to the monastery. There they learnt that no one had touched the bells, but that they had been set in motion by some miraculous power. Wonder and dismay came over all the pious people, and while they were still engaged in discussing the miracle a voice suddenly sounded forth among the clashing of the bells, clearer and more penetrating than any human voice, and the words were heard : ' I shall have pity on my people, O Mother.' These words were interpreted to imply that Mary's intercession had been granted by her Divine Son, and that the plague would abate within a short space." An immortal monument has been raised to St. Charles by Manzoni in his " Betrothed," but even without this the Italian people would not have allowed the memory of the great lover and saint to be forgotten. Of the many heroic ecclesiasts and saints who distinguished themselves during various epidemics of plague not one, with perhaps the exception of the legendary figure of St. Rochus, can be compared with him. Not only did he fearlessly visit the sick and dispense comfort everywhere, he sacrificed his whole fortune to his very bed to alleviate the needs of the poor. " Now on the approach of winter, when there was no provision to supply them with clothing and preserve them from the cold, but when the saintly kind-hearted father could not bear to see the poor suffering and did not know where to procure clothing for such large numbers, he ultimately hit on a good resource to collect all cloths in his household and have them cut up into many suits. With this means he seemed very satisfied and proceeded with it without delay. Thus he had his whole wardrobe and vestment chamber emptied, and cleared all the rooms of his palace of all cloths, curtains, tapestries, carpets, bed hangings, and such-like articles of material and cloth which were to be found in his establishment, and had them all made into clothes for the poor. It was a very curious and touching sight to see so great a crowd of poor people all dressed in the most various colours—some were in red, some in violet brown, some in green and other colours, as if they had been some beautifully arrayed army. When fitted out the whole procession betook themselves to the larger church of St. Ambrosius, to which the holy pastor had gone with bare feet, clad in so sad and miserable a garb that it moved everyone who saw him to deep compassion and loud weeping. Particularly as the man of God dressed in his long violet brown cardinal's robe, with train and hood, had pulled the hood, which usually hangs behind, over his head and down upon his eyes, and allowed the train which spreads out far behind and on the sides, and which, according to the custom of the Church, is usually carried after cardinals and potentates, to drag widely on the ground. But round his neck he had wound a great thick rope similar to the rope and noose which is usually placed round the neck of those condemned to die on the gallows. In his hands he bore a huge crucifix with the image of the Lord Jesus Christ fastened on it, which is to be seen at the present day in the cathedral. On this crucifix he fixed his eyes, bedewed with many tears, during the whole way immovably, as if he were He the Greatest of All, and like him as a criminal being led to public execution. For it has subsequently been ascertained that like Him he had sought to take all burdens and sins of his people upon himself and had offered himself to the Lord God as sacrifice, and had been prepared and willing to take upon himself the punishment of all sins, if only the divine wrath should be appeased against those who had deserved it, and the miserable town should be delivered from such vengeance and scourge. The sad and touching sight of their beloved father and holy shepherd awakened in the hearts of the Milanese such repentance and contrition that whilst the holy man was proceeding through to the streets in this guise the people broke into loud cries rising to heaven of ' *Misericordia, misericordia* ' ('Have mercy, God ; O Lord, have mercy'), as if each and every one's heart were about to burst with the pang of misery within his body. Which misery was still increased by the sight of all the cathedral clergy who, with bare feet and similarly mournful garb, took part in the procession. Alas! what a miserable procession it was. Alas ! what floods and torrents of tears fell on such a day. Since then the people of Milan have never beheld nor witnessed so wretched a sight."

As a true father of his people, Bishop Henri de Castel Moron de Belsunzo, who has been praised by Pope and Voltaire, proved himself during the plague at Marseilles. It was his merit that the despair of the unhappy town did not develop to complete disorganisation. Pope Clement VI assisted him in his pious work by issuing an extensive absolution for all those who dedicated themselves to the service of the sick. The moment has become celebrated when high up on the belfry of the church of Accoules, to the pealing of all the bells and the thundering of the guns of all the galleys in his diocese, he gave his benediction and, bowing to the four

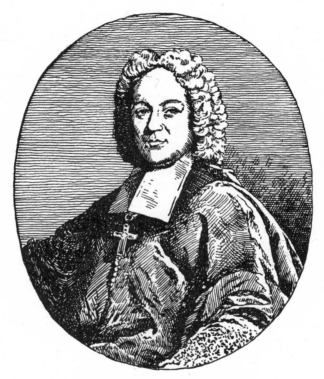

HENRI DE CASTEL MORON DE BELSUNZO.

points of the horizon, pronounced liturgical prayers, exorcising the plague.

It has already been mentioned that in times of plague great riches accrued to the Church. In the fourteenth century so much was given in the fear of death for the erection of altars, for bells and masses, that the Senate of Augsburg was obliged to take steps to secure some pittance for the rightful heirs. Koenigshoven, in his Strasbourg chronicle of 1381, remarks :

" Through this epidemic all the churches of Strasbourg became so rich that the old churches of St. Nicholas and St. Peter were pulled down and new roomy churches were erected." When in 1347 the plague was raging at Luebeck the confusion was so great that the citizens, as if deprived of their senses, took leave of life and willingly renounced all earthly possessions. They bore their treasures to the monasteries and churches to lay them on the steps of the altars. But for the monks the money had no attraction, for it brought death. They closed their gates, but the people threw their money over the walls of the monasteries; they would brook no impediment in their last pious work, to which they were urged by mute despair.

If we turn to the attitude of the Protestant Church we must first mention Martin Luther himself, who, during the various epidemics which visited Wittenberg in 1516, 1527, 1535, 1538, and 1539, was a shining example to his fellow citizens. When on August 25, 1527, the university was transferred to Jena on account of the plague prevailing at Wittenberg, he remained there as the only fellow of the University, together with Bugenhagen, the rector of the town. " My place is here," he declared, " and discipline forbids me to flee until such time when the same discipline may command. I hope that the heavens will not fall down if Frater Martinus should happen to die." It was in this most terrible time, 1527, that he wrote and composed the post powerful of his hymns—" A firm stronghold is our God." Of his fearless attitude, which bordered on temerity, we have various examples. Thus the wife of the burgomaster, Tilo Daene, nearly expired in his arms. When in 1526 the professor of law Sebald Muenster was carried off with his wife and three inmates of his house, upon which the students began to leave the town, Luther received the orphan children of Sebald in his house. " I have now survived three plagues," he once wrote, " and have visited some who were suffering from them, as in the case of Shadewalt, who had two plague boils ; I knew right well what they were, but it did me no harm; praise be to God ! That very time I came home and patted Margaret, who was then a little child, on the mouth without washing my hands. But truly I had forgotten it, otherwise I would not have done it, for it would be tempting God." He derides the timid student in a letter to the Elector: "I perceive that many of these young people lend a willing ear to all plague rumours, for some have blisters on their schoolbags, some a colic in their books, some scurvy in their pens and gout in their paper. Others find their ink mouldy, and others, again, have eaten their maternal letters and have in consequence been overcome by homesickness; and there are probably other ailments with which I am unacquainted." When, on October 22nd, he began to lecture on the twenty-second chapter of Genesis—several eminent persons had just died and Muenster had been buried the day before—his first words were: "*Non ideo lego quod cupiam vos hoc tempore hic retinere, quo timetur periculum pestiferæ luis. Quod si pestes imminet, fugiat qui volet, ac præcipue isti, qui sunt pavidi. Hos enim scriptura sancta jubet excedere castris, ne faciant pavere corda fratrum. Ego quidem grassantem luem hoc tempore non metuo, sed judico pavorem præcipuam huius mali causam esse.*" His pamphlet, "Is it Right to Flee from the Epidemic?" did much to appease the general confusion and panic. A few extracts may be quoted: "Nor is it necessarily a sign of small faith to fear death, which has been a terror to nearly all saints, and which is still a terror to them; and who would not praise those who are seriously so minded that they pay but little heed to death and submit willingly to the scourge of God? But, as with Christians, it is the case that there are but few strong and many weak, it can truly not be expected that all should bear the same burden. A man of strong faith may drink poison and it will not harm him, but one of weak faith would drink his death. St. Peter could walk upon the sea when his faith was strong, but when he doubted and became weak in faith he was about to drown. If a strong man walk with a weak one, truly he must adapt his pace to the strength of his companion, otherwise he would walk the weak man to death. But Christ does not desire that the weak should be cast aside, as St. Paul teaches us in the Epistle to the Romans, chapter xv, and in the 1st Epistle to the Corinthians, chapter xii"—"What is to be thought of those who having the plague secretly yet mix with the people? Answer: They are most wicked people who secretly having the plague mix with others, and they believe that if they can infect other people they would rid themselves of the infection and become sound—in this belief they go into the streets and enter the houses, so that they may pass on the plague to others or to their children and servants, and thus save themselves. And I truly believe that it is the devil who does this and helps to set the wheel in motion that this should be done. I am also told that some people are so desperately wicked that when infected with the plague they mix with other people, or go to their houses, because they are sorry that the plague is not there and desire to bring it there. Just as if this were the same kind of joke as if one were to put flies into anyone's room for fun. I do not know if I am to believe it, if it is true, then I do not know if we Germans are men or devils, it is true that there are exceedingly wicked people, and the devil is not slow to make use of them. In such cases I should advise that where such people are found the judge should seize them and hand them over to the executioner as real deliberate murderers and criminals. What else are such people but real murderers in the town ? Like murderers they stab a knife into one, and it is said that no one did it; thus they strike down here a child and there a woman, and it is said that no one has done it; and they go away laughing as if they had done something good. Thus it would be better to dwell with wild beasts than with such murderers. It is no use to preach to these murderers, they will not hear. I recommend to the authorities that they should remedy the matter, but not with advice and help of the physicians, but with that of the executioner. Has not God Himself ordained in the Old Testament that the lepers should be excluded from the congregation and should dwell outside the town; all the more we should do so in these dangerous epidemics, that if anyone is infected he should immediately isolate himself, or let himself be isolated from all others and immediately seek medical assistance; in this he should have assistance and not be forsaken in his need, so that the infection may be curbed in time, not only for the benefit of the one person, but of the whole community, which does not wish to be infected by it, as would be done if it were allowed to break out and spread to others. Thus our present plague is solely due to our negligence; the air, as yet, is still, praise be to God, fresh and pure, but some have been infected through temerity, and the Devil has his delight in the terror and flight which has broken out among us. May God prevent him. Amen!" Typical of Luther's delight in strong objective expressions is the epitaph which he composed for himself : "*Pestis eram vivus, moriens ero mors tua, Papa.*" "Alive I was thy plague, O Pope; when dying I shall be thy death."

Many writers inveighed against the flight of the rich, which gave rise to ill-feeling among the poorer classes. Nearly all reports of contemporaries agree in stating that the plague claimed most of its victims among the poor and badly nourished, for whom, as Simon de Couvino says, life itself was a kind of death. This bitterness was carried so far that the people in various towns of Italy believed that the plague had been artificially caused by the rich. Andreas Musculus, in his pamphlet, "Certain and Tried Physic against the Epidemic of Plague," 1561, emphatically denounces the rich who in times of need abandon their fellow citizens : " As in this recent epidemic we experienced how the children of the world were terrified at death, forsook home and belongings, and all half-dead with fear, pressed to the gates of the town to escape death and the epidemic, to prolong their lives and to continue to enjoy the delights and joys of the world. And on their return to resume even more intensely than before, like those who have escaped a heavy shower, in contempt of the Word of God, as they had done hitherto, the joys of this world, with scraping, grabbing, cheating, with ostentation and haughtiness. But, as the saying puts it : He who escapes his father falls into the hands of the judge. Thus, also, when the greatest among the rich who have been the main cause of God's wrath and have brought down this scourge and chastisement for the purpose of atonement, reformation, and redemption, immediately rush for the gate and do not at once feel the wrath of the scourge of God, and with unrepentant hearts once more return, as they had issued forth, and worse than ever before profiteer, scrape, grab, and display their wanton haughtiness, and even oppress the poor and believe there is no fear, as the catastrophe is over, and that they may enjoy the pleasures of life more intensely than before. But before they are aware, when God has chastened his own children and the number of the poor to bliss, he arouses Jack, the hungry peasant, and

Squire Plundersome, who, after shedding much blood, blocks the gates and beleaguers the town so that there is no escape. They take the town by assault, and God lets Jack slay and murder, break open the coffers with blunderbusses and halbards, and to measure with long lances what was brought in with short ells, scraped together against the Will of God and with an evil conscience; and this procedure has been observed by God since the creation of the world, that by means of brother Jack he visits and chastises those who have escaped his paternal, merciful scourge."

In the same pamphlet Musculus praises the Pomeranians and the maritime towns who, accustomed to epidemics, do not yield to heathen panics, but, placing their lives in the hand of God, quietly go on with their daily business without excess of dread or fear, saying, "He who is ripe let him fall."

We very frequently encounter in Protestant books of comfort and remedies invections against the "heathen, idolatrous atrocities of the Catholics," and particularly against the impotent plague idol as which they had established the pseudo-saint Rochus."

The title of a poem runs : "An approved medicine against the evils of the soul which cannot be obtained from Saints Sebastian or Rochus, but from the Lord Jesus Christ, the true Physician of Israel."

In reply to the question why in spite of the light of the Gospel there was such fear of the plague, Luther said that the lack of faith on the part of the people was one of the causes. "In popery the people relied on the merit of the monks and other things of that kind ; but now each one must look after himself and behave accordingly. Now, as with many, the faith and its resulting fruit is slight, the consequence is this dread of death."

Chants and hymns written in times of plague are numerous. Well known is "The Christian hymn composed by Huldrych Zwingli when he was seized by the plague." By far the most powerful hymns are : "How beautiful the morning star appears" and "Awake, a voice calls unto us," which Philip Nicolai wrote for his congregation during a terrible outbreak of plague at Unna in Westphalia.

APPENDIX

The Plague in the Monastery of St. Gall, a.d. 1629

Visitation of the Monastery of St. Gall by our most merciful Lord God in the year 1629

When on the 15th of October in the year 1628 the remains of Saints Othmar and Notker, as well as those of other patrons of the monastery, were solemnly transferred, it was believed that the monastery and town of St. Gall were threatened by the plague, which was prowling about here and there in the adjoining neighbourhood, and this fear was all the greater as great crowds of people came from the infected areas to the transference ceremony. But according to the design of God the All-Merciful, doubtless so that the honour of His saints should be preserved against the unjust railing of heretics, saying that the occasion of this ceremony had brought the plague into the country, the whole neighbourhood around remained free from infection. But it was different in the following year. The evil, fully deserved by our sins, began to break out in the town, to spread to the country, and to rage implacably in all quarters. At first it carried off our spiritual brothers, the parish priests of St. George and St. Fiden, so that consequently it became necessary—as no other parish priests were available—that at least one should go from our monastery to provide the infected with the last Sacraments. By order of our gracious Abbot Bernhard, the priests were summoned, so that their individual opinion might be heard. They all agreed that the people could not be abandoned without causing offence ; one or two who were able and willing to go should, therefore, be sent. There were some who would willingly have gone, but on account of age or decrepitude were unable, and perhaps there were also some who could have gone but did not wish to ; of those both willing and able to go there proved to be three : Father Deacon, Father Sub-Prior, and Father Kitchener (Archimagirus). Their readiness was reported to the gracious Abbot, but he was in doubt to whom he should in preference entrust this office. He brought the whole matter before the elders of the convention, who, in order to discuss the matter more freely, demanded the withdrawal of the candidates. On consultation they considered it not advisable to dispatch any one of the fathers in question, but were of opinion that the conditions of how those who were willing to undertake this service were to be treated should all be drawn up in writing. They believed that perhaps one or the other, when he became acquainted with these, would volunteer for the salvation of his fellow men. The conditions were drawn up and contained the following : Two, not one alone, were to be dispatched ; they were to live together with the others in one house, that for the celebration of Mass was to be provided with a portable altar ; there they were to have their necessary clothing, proper food, and service ; one of them was to hear confessions, and both be dispensed from the fasts imposed by the rule—a privilege seldom granted to the officials of the Church. Further, on their visits to the sick they were to enter no house, but to hear confessions outside, to bury no one, to dispense the Sacrament which was kept in their private house, but not the extreme unction, in the meanwhile to provide themselves with the necessary medicines, and while alive to enjoy special care in all cases of need, and after death the special comfort of intercession.

When these conditions had been read, however, no one volunteered, but the three above-mentioned fathers, who, in order to facilitate the discussion, again withdrew. They had declared that they could do no more useful and grateful service for God and for the monastery of St. Gall than by sacrificing their lives for the salvation of those entrusted to them. The designation of the individual persons was left to the Abbot. He delayed a long time. He was afraid to designate the Kitchener, as he had recently returned from curative treatment and might therefore be more easily susceptible to the plague. The whole question was therefore reduced to the Deacon and the Sub-Prior. At last he decided for the Sub-Prior, and gave him his paternal blessing. But he withdrew, I believe at the instigation of some other, his decision, and finally designated the Deacon, who was most zealous to obtain this office, and dismissed him with a benediction. He departed on the same day, after having previously taken leave of the priests and the younger brethren individually, and asked them to remember him in their prayers.   In the meanwhile a place was selected within and without the monastery where in any case those of the family or the monastery might be taken who should be infected with the plague.

Father Deacon had been fulfilling his office for a fortnight (he lived in the house of our steward, which bore the name of " Peartree "), and had hastened to assist both high and low, rich and poor, so that on the same day he frequently went out in various directions and visited eight, ten, twelve houses, till a secular priest arrived and relieved him of his onerous duties.   The Deacon returned to the monastery, but not to the convention.

In the meantime, whilst the Deacon was engaged outside in his duties, Father Augustine Rennhas, representative and custodian of our venerable head in the convention, began to sicken.   The doctor declared illness to be the so-called Hungarian fever, and entertained no hope for his recovery.   We therefore visited the good father, conversed with him, sat by his bed, sat up with him, gave the dying man the extreme unction, and were present when he expired and finally closed his eyes without thinking of any danger.   But when some undressed him they perceived upon his chest plague boils, which are called *pedechiæ*.   But they remained silent about this, either because they were not sufficiently acquainted with their signification or because they were afraid of causing a panic.   The deceased was therefore buried in the usual graveyard in the presence of the whole congregation, but with shorter ceremony than usual, lest delay and the sight of the corpse might prove dangerous to some.   For all were not without fear, particularly as on the previous day some belonging to the family of the monastery, as was known by some and surmised by others, had been infected by the plague.   These were a baker and a servant who had served the Father Deacon, who had returned to the monastery, but was away in the Palatinate, and, as they had been attacked by the prevailing disease, they had been taken to the presbytery of St. George, which had been set aside for this purpose.   But the servant went home, having either wrongly believed or stated that he was infected, and turned up in the monastery in good health after three days. These circumstances induced our gracious Abbot to decide on a change of residence for himself and to permit such change to all who desired to go elsewhere. He therefore issued an order that everyone was to write down whether he wished to remain or to go away. In reply to this all wrote, and there was indeed in nearly all so great a submission to the Will of God and their superiors that it is really worthy of being transmitted to posterity. I therefore quote the words which were written by each:

Father Deacon said: "I desire to remain here and serve those suffering from the plague both inside and outside the walls of the monastery, subject to the will of my superiors."

Father Sub-Prior said: "I desire to remain here during this sad time of plague, unless it be the will of my superiors that I should not."

Father Bartholomæus wrote: "Father Bartholomæus will remain. God's Will be done."

Father Ulrich wrote: "Above all I wish to be obedient to our gracious Abbot, after that my wish is to remain here."

Father Kilian wrote: "I should prefer to remain at St. Gall and labour for the salvation of souls, if this be pleasing to my gracious Abbot; to whose decision I submit entirely, and whose orders in this matter I humbly await; I am more desirous of being led and ordered than of leading and ordering."

Father Marian wrote: "I will remain here if it is not contrary to the orders of my superiors."

Father Justus wrote: "After mature consideration and prayer for the grace of the Holy Ghost, I should like to remain here under the present circumstances for the benefit of my own salvation and that of my fellowmen, and with the benediction of Your Highness I shall, if Your Grace and my other superiors consider me capable of doing something either in or outside of the monastery, obey joyfully; but as on account of the sickness from which I have just recovered, and which does not appear to be entirely healed, I have not complete confidence in myself. I therefore leave it to the decision of my superiors and of the physician. For the rest may the Will of God be done with me."

Father Benedict wrote : "Brother Benedict desires for certain reasons, which are known to his superiors, to go away."

Father Hieronymus wrote : "Brother Hieronymus wishes to remain."

Father Anton wrote : "Gracious Lord Abbot, although up to the present I have not been of robust health, and am somewhat afraid of the epidemic, I have nevertheless resolved, after fervent prayer for the grace of the Holy Ghost and after supplication for the protection of the Virgin Mary, to whom I am entirely devoted, to remain (should Your Grace not wish it otherwise) with St. Gall, St. Othmar, St. Notker, and our other patrons, if it is possible for me to be of any service."

Father Beat said : "I submit to holy obedience; may that which is the Will of God and my superiors be done."

Father Constantinus wrote : "As at the moment I can see no reason for a change of place, I have resolved in confidence in the Divine providence to remain here, if this should be agreeable to my Lord Abbot."

Father Mansuetus wrote : "Gracious Lord Abbot! In confidence in the assistance of God and of the saints, I will remain in the monastery of St. Gall, if such be the will of Your Grace."

Father John wrote : "Gracious Lord Abbot! Should Your Grace consider it preferable that I should remain here, I will do so willingly, otherwise I am much afraid of the plague."

Father Placidus wrote : "I will remain here, if my superiors do not desire it otherwise."

Father Bonaventura wrote : "As after close observation of my character I find that I am somewhat timid and am unable to see of what use I could be for the salvation of souls if I were to remain at St. Gall, I most humbly and sincerely request Your Highness to permit me to change my residence. But whatever Your Grace may command I will willingly execute."

Father Michael wrote: "Most Reverend Father, in regard to the present misfortune I was always of the convinction and opinion that not only should I not go away, but, by the help of God, with all my forces do service and give assistance to others. But, as I do not possess sufficient strength to serve the people outside, as I am not strong enough to go about either on horseback or on foot, and my debility is so great that with the best intention I could not do it, I have resolved day and night in the confessional to exert my full powers (should I be considered worthy to do it), and if Your Grace desires it, and necessity demands it, without regard to my debility, for the sake of God, of the souls and my obedience, to serve outside those stricken with the plague. As far as it depends on me, I have no desire to remove to any other place. As, however, it is not only a question of me, but of my brethren, I humbly request Your Reverence that, should it be in accordance with your wise decision to dismiss the young also, not to send them out into the world, at least not those who are about to enter on their novitiate. But in this also I submit to Your Grace "

So far the opinions expressed by the priests now follow those of the younger brethren :

Brother Othmar places himself entirely at the will and disposal of his superiors, " ready to live and to die, as is the Will of the Lord ; let him do what in his eyes seems good, in the first place may the will of heaven be done. After that, if it can be done without any harm, I desire to remain with my preceptor and my younger brethren either in life or death. Whether this desire is of the spirit or the flesh (the latter I should like to exclude entirely from consideration) I leave to the decision of my superiors."

Brother Carolus wrote : " I (if I am to speak according to my heart) wish to remain at St. Gall, and if I am capable of any service I should like to render it to my brethren or others. But I place myself entirely under the orders of my superiors, and shall remain content with anything they may be pleased to do."

Brother Athanasius wrote : " I am ready to do anything my superiors may desire, although, if it depended on me, I should prefer to remain here, as I have selected the place as my residence. Let the Will of God and my superiors be done. I am resigned; so that what my superiors decide is, as it should be, for me the most agreeable."

Brother Chrysostomos wrote : "I place myself quite at the disposal of Your Grace, submit myself entirely into the hands of Your Grace ; whatever the gracious Abbot may decide in regard to me I consider the best, for I fear nothing but trust firmly in the power of God and the protection of our saints."

Brother Ignatius wrote : " I submit myself to the protection of Your Grace, and more particularly to that of God and our guardian angels."

Brother Basilius wrote: " I will remain here, if Your Grace considers it good that I should."

Brother Gallus wrote : " I will go away or remain, as is considered best by my superiors ; to me it is a matter of indifference."

Brother Bonifacius wrote : " I submit myself entirely to Your Grace and surrender myself into your hands; whatever you do I shall consider best. I am prepared to go away if it pleases Your Grace, as I do not see under the present circumstances of what use I can be."

Brother Desiderius wrote : " I submit myself humbly to Your Grace and surrender myself into your hands, whatever you consider best, to that I shall agree. But if it depended on me I would be a hundred, yea a thousand fold, submissive to my superiors here."

After having read all these expressions of opinion the gracious Abbot resolved to go to Rorschach and to take the younger brethren with him, to send the two priests who wished to go away to Wil, and to leave the rest in the name of God at St. Gall.

Although the physician would have preferred that the gracious Abbot should have gone to Wil so that he should not have been exposed to danger by the young people, who were particularly susceptible to the plague, in the meanwhile he refused to flee any further than Rorschach. There he proceeded on September 5th, having ordered the younger brethren to follow next day with Father John Geiger, professor of philosophy, who was to be their future instructor.

There was a considerable fuss as to what was to be done with the pupils; finally it was decided that those who could shortly enter on their novitiate should go to Rorschach, and that the others should be sent home. Thus, on September 11th six of them, Jacob Nussbomer, Theodor Bridler Matthias

Negelin, Jacob Karrer, Balthasar Huwiler, Matthew Hertenstein, together with their preceptor, Michael Widemann,
were sent to Rorschach. As seventh they were accompanied
by Marcus Leemann, who, on account of prevalence of plague
at Gossau, could not be sent home. The others were sent
home two days later : Henry Buntener to Uri, George Henry
of Waldkirch to Rheinau, Caspar Pfister to Marchdorf, Theodor
Reding to the monastery near Rorschach, and, finally, Hieronymus Pfaw to Ueberlingen. But as the two latter were in the
same school standard as the candidates for the novitiate,
when they arrived at Rorschach they were received in the
monastery. Among the pupils there had been two wards of
our venerable Head, Christian Fortunatus and Jeremias
Brouder. These two slept in the dormitories, attended all
religious services with us, waited at table, read aloud, and did
everything they were told to do. When one of them was
observed on September 15th by the Deacon, who had returned
to the convention on the 11th of the month, to be eating and
drinking nothing at dessert, he was questioned, and confessed
that at breakfast he had been seized by a dislike for the egg
dish, which had grown cold, and that while cleaning the
dormitory he had felt a headache. Father Deacon, fearing
something serious, gave him some *aqua theriacalis* to drink
and made him sweat. He sweated in the upper dormitory,
but he vomited the medicine. Next day he was ordered to
go down to the lower dormitory of the pupils. There again
he began to sweat, but there were no clear indications of the
plague. Nevertheless, by order of the Deacon, he remained
in the schoolroom and prepared for confession. When on
the third day, quite early in the morning, the poison had broken
out in plague boils, he confessed, took communion, and was
taken to St. George's.

On the same day Father Placidus was laid up. He had
previously taken medicine, and as this always disagreed with
him, so it did this time. He complained of cold, vomited,
had a dislike for food and drink, and was obliged to remain in
bed. We were inclined to attribute his sickness to the medicine, visited him, sat by his bed, and were not afraid of making
it up, all the more so as in his serene humour, indicative of the
highest degree of patience, he joked with us about his sickness,

which he called a whim. When I was making up his pillow for him he said : " Oh, let me lie hard, so that I may at least suffer something for the honour of God." However, being anxious about the salvation of his soul, he resolved to be prepared for any danger and provided with the Holy Sacraments. But as on account of the dryness of his throat he did not venture to take Holy Communion, he stated, after confession, that what he most ardently desired was to be fortified by the Last Sacrament; but as he could not do this without disrespect he would for greater honour to God refrain from it. The doctor was sent for. He visited the patient in his cell, and, although he did not quite like the look of him, he did not care to hint at plague, or to recommend a change of place. " As we know," he said, " that the cause of sickness is to be found in the medicine, which is repugnant to him, we will leave him till to-morrow and see how he is." But it was inconvenient to nurse him in his bedroom, and we decided to move him to the perspiring-room of the Preceptor just opposite his own room. He was taken across while we were at dinner. Father Deacon examined him and found on his arms and chest signs of plague boils. He therefore prepared for certain death, and received extreme unction from Father Bartholomæus. When he was asked if he would not move into the schoolrooms (for the women's quarters had already been prepared for this purpose), he replied: "Put me wherever you want; I will willingly lie on the ground outside." He asked us to edify him with prayers treating of faith, hope, and love. Whilst I was praying to him he repeated the words with intense devotion, and assured me that he gladly sacrificed his young life, which perhaps he might have preserved by flight, to God, he had nothing on earth that attracted him, and hoped to be in heaven on the morrow. This he repeated subsequently frequently, although soon terrible heart spasms and dying qualms caused him to utter loud screams. We were anxious to know how we were to convey him to the schoolroom. Then he said himself : " You must not carry me, I will walk myself." When I asked if he would be able to, he said : " I will run quickly." The sick attendant leading him by the hand, and I, together with the Father Deacon accompanying him, holding a light (the day was just breaking), he walked manfully to the room set aside for those infected. At the gate of the monastery I bid my dear brother farewell, for the Deacon instructed me to go and order the fathers who lived near to his bedroom to move their quarters. Father Deacon, together with the Steward, led him to the school quarters. When on his way he passed the visitors' quarters, and fathers and brothers, weeping, expressed good wishes for him, he wished them all good night and asked to be remembered in their prayers. Father Deacon went with him at some distance to the school quarters, and gathered from his conversation, among other things, that when offering the Sacrament to a boy, Lucas Karrer, whose father had died of the plague, a violent shivering fit had seized him, and he had felt a boil, but that this had disappeared again, so that it was thus doubtful how he had come by the plague. It is certain that first he stayed a long time with Father Augustin before his death, and then heard that it was quite uncertain if he was to remain or go away, and he felt very nervous, particularly during the night, so that he had asked his neighbour if he woke up in the night to give a sign by coughing or clearing his throat that this might dispel his terrors. About eight o'clock the Deacon left him, when he was very composed and quite resigned to the Will of God, and in addition comforted that he was dying in the good work of obedience. The Deacon hardly entertained any hope, although the sick attendant was of a different opinion, that he would survive the next day. At about eleven o'clock at night his life terminated, as we trust in a blissful end. Next day, in the early morning, he was borne by the sick attendant alone to St. Peter's, as none of the servants dared to give assistance. It was, indeed, difficult to find people who would dig a grave. When finally he was buried he was deemed happy by some to have deserved in life to rest in so holy a place after his death.

Early the same day, September 18th, Father Deacon (perhaps he had been somewhat negligent the day before) felt a roughness in his throat, and on his neck a hard place and a swelling, but it did not pain him. He took stapediana and sweated. After breakfast he walked out into the country with the others, but was not very lively; but he did not appear at dinner, as if, on account of stomach trouble, he was unable to eat anything he might have easily aroused suspicion of sickness in others. Instead of his meal he again took stapediana, and, as his stomach refused it, *aqua theriacalis*, sweated slightly, and felt rather chilly. I knew about all this, and informed Father Stewart. We two resolved to write to the doctor to come in that night and visit the sick father at a distance. He came at our request about nine o'clock, aroused the shivering man, and talked to him not at a distance but quite close. He felt his pulse, even felt the swelling on his neck with his hand, and did other things which surprised us. He announced that, as there were indications of plague, Father Deacon should be isolated, but, as the hour was inconvenient, it should be left to the decision of the patient himself whether he would go out of the monastery that night. We informed Father Deacon, who, in reply to all, said he was quite ready to go away if before he went he was given extreme unction. Father Bartholomæus was called, who anointed the sick man kneeling in the church. About eleven we conducted him to the school dormitory, the dying man comforting us who were weeping, and finally asking us to bestow our blessing on him, and in the name of the Abbot to give him the assurance of being permitted to sacrifice his life in the fulfilment of obedience. Thus he went up the stairs, down which he was never to come, to the first schoolroom, which was still clean, as Father Placidus had expired in the upper story.

Very early in the morning I dispatched Father Stewart to Rorschach to inform the gracious Abbot of the sad incident and to bring back orders as quickly as possible what was to be done with the rest of the convention. All the rooms had been infected, and some of the fathers appeared to be very anxious. Very soon, in the course of a few hours, he returned and reported the decision of the gracious Abbot. Those who were nervous were to name the place where they wished to go, and the others who desired for the honour of God and the salvation of their fellow men to remain in the convent were to select quarters where they chose to live. There were four who wished to go away—the Fathers Marianus, Antonius, Beatus, and Mansuetus; eight who wished to remain—the Fathers Bartholomæus, Udalricius, Notkerus, Kilianus, Justus (who first consulted the doctor as to whether, on account of his illness, contracted at Fulda, he would be particularly prone to the plague, to which he received a negative reply), Hieronymus, Constantinus, and Pius. The former were ready to go anywhere the Abbot might order, the latter decided to move to the house known by the name of " Hell " and the buildings above the Abbey. All this was decided before breakfast. During breakfast it was remarked by some that Father Mansuetus did not seem very well—he was neither eating nor drinking, and appeared to be losing his sight ; in short, he seemed to be infected. I called the father out (as nearly all were taking medicine, we did not dine at our usual table), questioned him; he confessed what it was. Although he did not believe that the disease had developed so far, at the exhortation of the elders he proceeded with many tears to the school quarters, being led by me and Father Bartholomæus, and occupied a room which was still pure and uninfected. When, after a few weeks, he was again restored, he assured that he had gone in great fear, but so soon as he had been up there he set aside all anxiety.

I immediately sent the Steward to Rorschach to report to the gracious Abbot what we had decided before breakfast, and to bring news what further orders he wished to issue. The Abbot ordered the three fathers who wished to go to Wil were to be sent to Father Jodocus (as was done the following day), and that those who were remaining were to move into the buildings mentioned, which they did on the same day, September 19th—Ulrich and Kilian going to the quarters above the Abbey, which are known by the name of the sweating-room or " Hell " ; the adjoining rooms being taken by Bartholomæus, Justus and Constantinus, the Capuchin sweating-room by the Sub-Prior, the Steward and the Kitchener remaining in their cells. The so-called centre sweating-room we used as a refectory. At first we excluded the servants of the monastery, and ordered that only those should be admitted within the gates who were free from suspicion of infection. We fulfilled the holy obligations of our foundation and our duties as monks in these sad times in the following manner: The daily death vigil was entrusted to the young brethren and pupils at Rorschach shortly after their departure ; the Virgin Mass, together with the Saint Anne Mass and the weekly

Mass for departed souls, we entrusted to the perceptors of the young. But we soon reclaimed the Virgin Mass for St. Gall on the urgent advice of pious fathers, who hoped that under the protection of the Blessed Virgin we should be safer. The so-called Chapel Mass and the Daily Mass or Gate Mass were taken over by the fathers who were going to Wil, who, however, neglected to fulfil the obligation, so that on their return they had to make good for their neglect.

Thus we remained free of every obligation except those incumbent on the choir. At first, when the plague began to appear, here and there we had, in accordance with the wish and advice of the elder fathers, taken over three Masses a day— the first at the High Altar, the second at the altar of St. Othmar, and the third at the altar of St. Notker to obtain the protection of our saints, but voluntarily and without any obligation; and had read these Masses up to this time in so far as it had been possible without inconvenience. But as the number of priests decreased no one was appointed to read them, which was probably to our disadvantage, for, according to the observation of some, Father Placidus and our cleric Christian began to sicken with the plague from that Saturday on which these Masses were abolished. We therefore subsequently as often as possible made up for these Masses. Further, we went for the day and night hours from our quarters to the church. We chanted High Mass and Vesper and prayed the other hours, the shorter ones at six o'clock, so that from that time it was more convenient to read Mass and to hear the confessions of the people. These came flocking in crowds, so that we could hardly satisfy all. We often went fasting to the Confessional (so that afterwards we might read Masses in the presence of the people), and confessed those crowding up from all sides (God knows how many infected there were among them). But as later on the danger increased, it was forbidden to hear confession fasting, therefore all Masses were read early. On Sundays and Feast Days only one Mass was read, and this one not in the choir but at the altar of the Holy Cross.

The people did not take Communion at this altar, but at the one opposite, and often in such numbers (on account of the quantity of deaths) that Communion was finished long after Mass. In addition, on Sundays and Feast Days the

Most Holy in the monstrance was exhibited outside the choir as a substitute for the omitted Mass and the Catechism, and to stimulate greater piety and more zealous faith in the minds of the believers. At the termination of the Compline every day after the Angelus a sign was given with the larger bell to exhort the people on hearing it to say five paternosters with extended arms, together with the creed to the honour of the five wounds of Christ, to drive away the plague. After the sounding of the bell, we remained in the choir, each one in his place, and carried out an examination of conscience for a quarter of an hour. At last, having been warned to avoid the harmful night air, we began to celebrate the Compline after Vespers, and the morning prayers each one in his cell. The prescribed fasts, abstinence from meat, we observed on Monday, Wednesday, and Friday. We could not have a regular dinner, and therefore had to dispense with the customary readings, but at first a cleric and later a Frater Conversus used to read to us at dessert. While all this was going on various fates were meted out to our patients. So far as Christian was concerned, no one doubted that he would recover, although he was very ill; also all believed that the Deacon would certainly escape. He was active and serene, often wanted to go out for a walk and read Mass. But the doctor would not permit it. But the Sacrament was brought to him, so that he might celebrate Communion for himself. Father Mansuetus, it was unanimously believed, would not last long. Of this we were so confident that a general council was held in which a burial-place was determined for the deceased. By Father Deacon he was provided with the Last Sacraments, and it was believed that he would not survive the night. But God changed his fate. Christian began to recover gradually, and when his health was completely restored he was once more received in the monastery.

Father Mansuetus also began, whilst remaining in bed most of the time, to feel stronger every day and to conceive hope of recovery. At last he attained it, but was before recovery much tormented with gout and rheumatic pains. For the first time he celebrated Mass on the festival of St. Gall, the second time in the chapel of St. Catherine, and four days later he returned to our usual sick-room. On All

Saints' Day he heard confession again in our church, and was again in the company of the other fathers.

On the other hand, Father Deacon, who had taken most medicines prescribed by the anxious doctor, as by their effect his throat was swollen and he combated a boil which had developed on his neck by scorpion oil, began on the eighth day of his illness to feel worse, for the poison had struck inwardly. He sweated, had headache, took a loathing for his food, and wandered in his talk. Finally, plague boils appeared on the chest—generally a certain indication of death. He was already sure that he was going to die, and assured the doctor of it. But the latter did not weary of trying to find some means of saving his friend. He hoped to attain this if the boils would burst with the plague sweat and the poison find a way out from the interior. For this purpose he sent him immediately very expensive medicines, which he prepared with great care with his own hands; but, alas! all in vain. The immortal physicians Kosmus and Damianus were more powerful than the mortal physician. Just on the day of their festival the excellent father felt that he must relinquish this mortal life. He therefore dispatched early in the morning the sick attendant to the Sub-Prior: he was about to pass to eternal life, if he were happy he would bear us all in mind; he requested (as he had already done two days before) to bid farewell in his name to the gracious Abbot and all fathers and brethren; he asked them to forgive his faults and to pray for the deceased. He also begged to be remembered to the fraternity of the Most Blessed Virgin and to the congregations of the neighbouring monasteries. Finally, he requested that his old linen undergarment and other things necessary for burial should be sent him; for the purpose of enveloping in them his dying limbs while he was still alive, and thus to deck himself with his own hands for his marriage with the Lamb. With reluctance we sent what he demanded (who could do it with indifference), but he continued to ask for the clothing. At last he received it. Then raised himself in his bed, put on his vest and drew the linen garment round, but as he fainted he was only completely clothed by the servants. In the convention it was not known that the father was in extremities, but when the Sub-Prior heard it from the door-

keeper he immediately went to him with the Kitchener to
bid him farewell if he could only cast a glance through the
window. He immediately slipped out of his bed, and pulled
himself with the help of the servants to the window and
looked out quite pale and feeble : " I first thought that my
eyes were deceiving me.   Forgive me my faults and pray for
me." When the fathers wished to engage in further conversation and asked for his blessing, he begged them to dismiss
him as he could no longer remain out of his bed.   Hardly had
he returned when with prayers, in which he joined with heart
and mouth, he expired while the servants invoked the most
holy names of Jesus and Mary according to his instructions.
After sunset he was interred in the new churchyard near to
the place of St. Othmar. We had previously resolved to
bury him in the chapel of St. Peter, but, as it was his wish to
rest by the side of St. Othmar, this wish was fulfilled. His
death was deeply regretted by the Lord Abbot. To a
witness of his grief, Father John, who stood near him,
he said repeatedly : " Alas, dearest Brother, what a honest
and useful man we have lost ! We have lost our most beloved
Father Deacon," and further words to that effect. The day
before he, as we hoped, entered heaven ; Father Deacon had sent
thither in advance, as we confidently trust, Frater Conversus
Egger, a man of the best reputation and life. Four days
before he had fallen ill here.   At first he believed to be suffering
from something else, but isolated from the others and brought
into a little house used by the Conversing Brethren for
bathing, he drove by means of sweat-inducing medicines the
poisons out, and expired duly provided with the Last Sacraments
on September 26th about two o'clock inspired with the best
hope.

In the night preceding the death of the Deacon one of our
older servants, a man called Schaffhausen, was on night duty
in the monastery.   Before midnight he had carefully announced
the hours, but in the early morning, seized by a certain terror,
without thinking of illness, he had gone home.   After a few
hours he sent to our cellar master requesting white bread and
wine, but he did not mention that he was ill, and said he
would return to the monastery next day.   But having said
this in the morning, he was a corpse by the afternoon.

It may easily be seen that all the rooms of the convention, indeed of the whole monastery, were infected.

Another servant, a carter, was seized with the plague and taken to St. George, where in the space of three days he died. To the same place they took our cleric, Hieremias, who had been our partner at meals, and who had read to us. In him the plague had produced in the course of three days so high a degree of madness that, as he was locked up in his room and could escape in no other way, he jumped out of the window and ran into the neighbouring wood. From there he was fetched back on the 30th of September, about nine o'clock in the evening, and died.

Whilst all this was happening at St. Gall quiet prevailed at Rorschach, and the young people established there were once more reduced to discipline. As a protection against the plague they said daily the litany of St. Othmar, together with other prayers, and before going to bed they sang in the chapel Notker's " *Media Vita*," together with the Lauretanian litany. But it was the will of God that this monastery should also suffer visitation. Of the pupils who had recently left St. Gall two, as was stated above, were received at Rorschach : Theodore Reding and Hieronymus Pfaw. With these, or at least with their bedding, it is believed the infection was introduced. If in the bed of one of these, before it was sent to Rorschach, Christian, who was infected, had slept and sweated, as has been maintained, it was Theodor's bed, and he first caught the plague from the bed and developed signs of it. As at first these were doubtful and uncertain, the pedagogue and preceptor, Father Michael, had no compunction in going to him himself, and even examining and feeling the painful spot. The illness was reported to his father. He sent an old peasant who knew nothing about the matter to examine the boy. He did so, and said there was no question of plague. When he was told to go home, he changed his mind and said the boy was infected. He was therefore sent to the country, to the home of his parents. He was bathed in tears, not so much on account of the fear of death as on account of the sad separation from his comrades. After his departure Hieronymus was slightly affected by illness, which he could no longer conceal. The matter was reported to the Lord Abbot with full details, and he ordered that all the boys should be sent home. When they were told this, weeping and wailing pervaded the whole monastery, as they found it hard to leave us. But as all could not well be sent to their parents, as they would have to have been sent to plague-stricken districts, four of them—Matthew Nagelin, Theodor Bridler, Balthasar Huwiler, and Matthew Hertenstein —were sent, at the urgent request of the Brothers of Murbach, to the Revisors of Murbach. But they were not admitted into the monastery immediately on account of the danger, but retained a few days at Gebwill Castle.

After their disposal Father Michael, who up to then had lived apart with the boys, wished to rejoin the other brothers and to participate in their common meals. But he was advised to delay a little longer and to remain in his room, so that there should be no risk of his spreading the disease, which he might have caught from the boys. This advice was sound—although Father Michael did not know that he had caught the infection from Theodor and was secretly developing it—he obeyed, and held aloof from the society of the others. On the same day, September 27th, which proved so fatal for Father Deacon, he took some pills which the doctor had prescribed for him as an autumnal treatment ; but their effect was so disastrous, as the medicine, by stirring up the poison which until then had lain latent, caused a plague boil to break out in the vicinity of his genitals, but without causing him pain. He therefore held his peace and made no complaint. After breakfast, so as not to be alone, he sent word to Father John that he wished to have conversation with one or two brothers to while away the time. The latter, suspecting no ill, dispatched two, Carolus and Basilus. Hardly had they been engaged in conversation for an hour when suddenly Father Michael was seized with shivering fits, followed by fever and violent headache. He felt it was the plague, and broke off the conversation, dismissed the brothers, and ordered them to summon Father John. The latter came immediately, but was not admitted into the room by the patient, who informed him that he was infected by the plague, and would talk to him in the open air.

Father John agreed, and arranged for an interview in the

upper orchard. He went on first, Father Michael followed him, limping slightly on account of his boil. When they reached the appointed place he immediately informed him of the nature of his disease, and expressed a desire to confess and prepare himself for certain death. Father John, feeling fraternal sympathy with the sick man, encouraged and comforted him, seeking to minimise the indications and nature of the disease, and saying that it had not come so far yet that he needed to fear the proximity of death. It was probably only " vanishing boils," he said, which break out suddenly and then disappear again. But as Father Michael complained of intolerable burning in his head and extraordinary thirst, he plucked a bunch of ripe grapes from a vine and gave them to the sick father to eat. The good father accepted the gift, but after having eaten one or two of the grapes he felt an inclination to vomit. " Alas ! I cannot eat them; what a pity for the grapes, where shall I throw them away ? " When Father John showed him a nettle patch, he refused to throw the bunch into it, and said : " Someone might find it and in eating it come by his death." He therefore went a little ahead of his companion and threw it beneath the little bridge into the flowing brook. Then he returned and begged Father John (his usual confessor) to hear his general confession.

The latter promised to do so, and fixed as time four o'clock in the afternoon, and as place the orchard in which they were. At the time agreed both came to the place arranged. The patient confessed kneeling on the ground, with upraised hands, quite overcome and penitent. Father John did not listen at a distance, but, prompted by love, quite close to him. When he had spoken comfort to the penitent, he also gave him something for his physical complaint—*aqua theriacalis*, which he ordered him to take so that he might be made to sweat.

All this was carried out in secret—no one knew anything about it, except Father John, who for that night intentionally kept silent, either so as not to cause fear to the others, or because he hoped that the medicine would cure the patient. They waited for the next day. Then Father Michael, early in the morning, sent a note to Father John reporting with rejoicing that he had quite recovered, was feeling no more pains but quite well, and requesting to be allowed to read Mass. Father John suspected some ill from the treacherous nature of the infection, which frequently conceals itself for a time to break out again with greater vehemence. He refused his request, and forbade him to go out in the open air, and besought him in the meanwhile to remain in his room. But piety and too great confidence in his health induced Father Michael not to heed this advice. He read his Mass, prayed, and went through all functions like a healthy man. After breakfast he was unexpectedly again assailed by an attack of the plague, he was seized with fever, and felt himself worse than ever. He wrote to Father John, describing his sad condition much in this manner: "I see, alas! I see and feel distinctly, that I am really suffering from the plague—I am shivering all over my body, shaking with cold, and suffer from nausea. My case must be reported to the Sub-Prior at St. Gall. Take my urine to the physician that he may devise some antidote to help me. I wish to write several other things, but the trembling and shaking of my limbs prevents me." Father John without delay informed the Steward and the other elders in the house of the incident, and sent news to the physician and the Sub-Prior at St. Gall. The former sent the good father spiritual comfort in a letter full of cordial sympathy, and the latter a medicine to be taken at nightfall, one of the strongest with which he was acquainted. Of this sad case the Abbot was so far unaware, for no one would undertake or dared to report it to the weak old man. Finally he heard of it in the following manner. It was at the evening celebration of the festival of St. Michael, at supper-time. While supper was going on a note written by Michael was brought, in which he once more asked for Father John as confessor. The latter informed the company of the matter. They advised him not to go, and to await the decision of the Abbot in the matter. Father John, undecided, reported the whole matter to the Abbot. He, very much perturbed at the unhappy incident in the house, urged that either the parish priest or the steward, if he were not afraid of the plague, should go to confess the patient. The steward undertook to go that same evening, and placed a very bright light between himself and the patient; next morning, with the same precaution, he administered communion to him. Upon this Father John sent for three brothers from Murbach, Benedict, Simperus, and Deicolus, frankly disclosed to them the dangers of the plague, and advised them to consider if they would remain there or return home. All considered, and came to the resolution to remain with the brethren of St. Gall, saying : " They were afraid that if they proceeded to Murbach they would be retained there and not allowed to continue their studies. They hoped the superiors would consider them as brethren of St. Gall and transfer them to a place of safety."

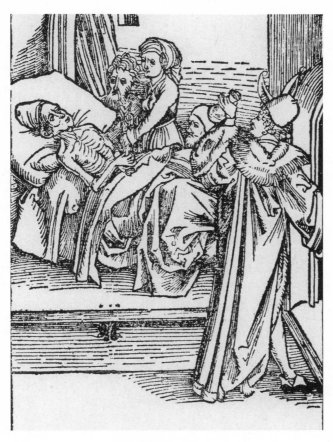

THE DOCTOR'S VISIT
Anonymous woodcut from Geiler von Kaisersperg's
Ship of Fools, 1520

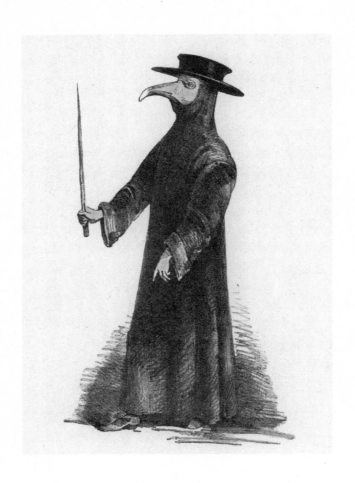

THE BEAK DOCTOR
From the *Historiae anatomicae*
by Thomas Bartholin (Hafniae 1661)

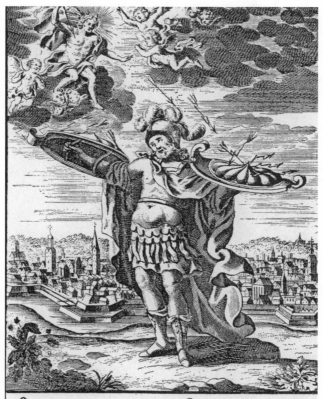

Sagittæ potentis acutæ in Sebastianico confrin-
guntur scuto.

Die pfeil deß erzürneten Gottes stoßen sich ab
an den Sebastianischen schild.

VITA ET GESTA SANCTI SEBASTIANI AUGSPURG
Etching from Hemer, 1702

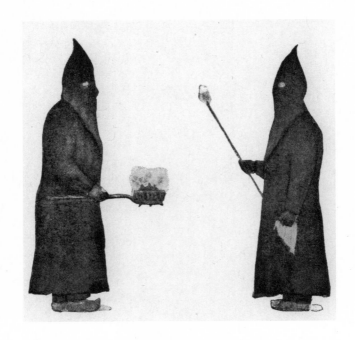

Sick attendants during the plague of Marseilles, 1720

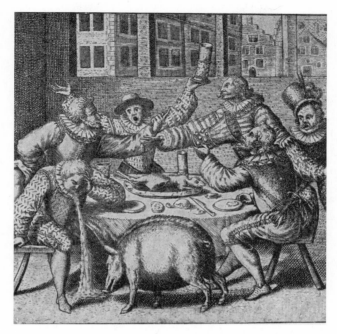

Ebrietas et Luxus [Drunkeness and Excess]
by Theodor de Bry (1528–98)

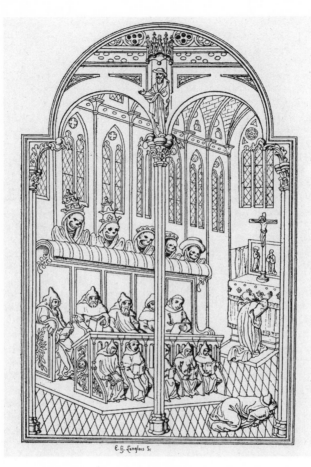

French Minature from the Psaltry of Henry VI (1431)

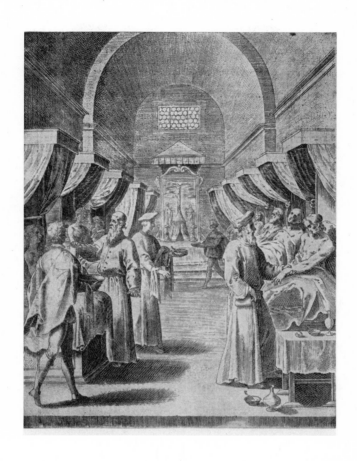

Hospital Sancti Joannis, Roma, 1588

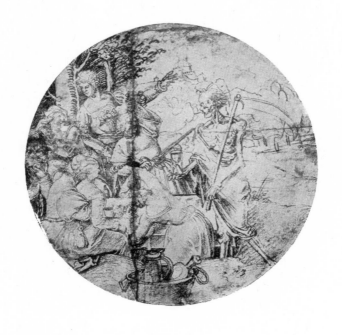

COMPANY AND DEATH
by Hans Baldung Grien (1470–1522)

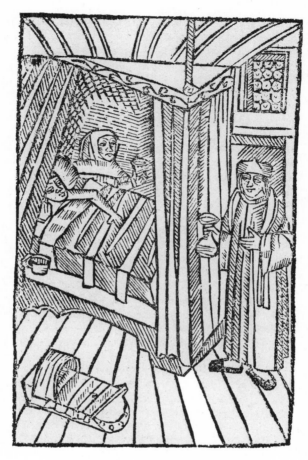

MARRIED COUPLE SICK OF THE PLAGUE
from *Vur die Pestilentz*, Cologne, 1508

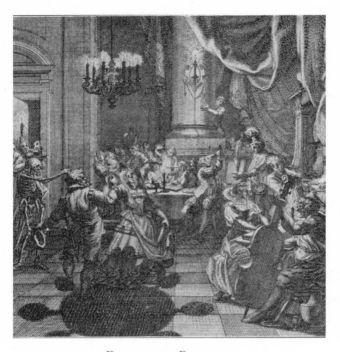

DEATH IN THE BALLROOM
Etching by Michael Rentz (1701–58)

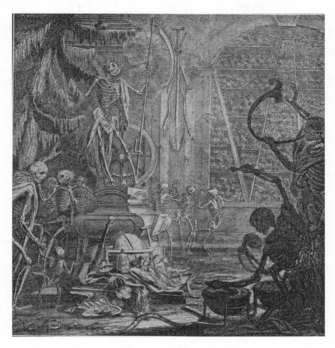

DANCE OF DEATH
Etching by Michael Rentz (1701–58)

CHAPTER VII

THE DIABOLIC ELEMENT IN THE PLAGUE

Devil worship—Moral collapse of the Church—The Luciferians—Robber bands—Liberated galley slaves—The plague-house steward and his gang—Domination of the rabble—Gravediggers as angels of death—Bestial violation of the living and the dead—The inferno of the hospitals—The plague kiss of the scholar—Artificially spread plague—Diabolic mummies—Suspected Lutherans—The Milan plague-makers' trial—A diabolical vision—Legacy hunters spread the plague—Cruel law courts.

In the fourteenth century not only the Dance of Death originated under the impression of the plague, but also the bas-relief sculptures in the cathedrals which represent human figures kneeling before the Devil and doing homage. For diabolic wickedness, particularly the period after 1350, as is already pointed out by Johannes von Mueller, may be compared with the times of the Atrides in heathen antiquity. " On the conclusion of the Holy Year the lords of the towns and castles resumed their feuds, the morals deteriorated. Sensuality alone prevailed ; justice and pity were powerless, so soon as it appeared advantageous to murder or poison rivals in power at the hospitable board. The science of finance was reduced to robbery, politics to perjury ; they were less efficient in the use of arms in the field than in their use for assassination." The religious discipline and piety of the mediæval ages had long ago yielded to the unrestricted arbitrariness of the individual, and the Church itself had become degenerate. The Minor Friar Johannes of Winterthur and the Westphalian Dominican Heinrich of Herford have left a terrible testimony for the years 1348 and 1349 :

" How contemptible the Church has grown, especially in its most important representatives, who lead a bad life and have sunk even deeper than the others. For the shepherds of the Church feed themselves instead of their flocks, these they shear or rather fleece ; their conduct is not that of the shepherd but of the wolf ! All beauty has vanished from the Church of God; from head to toe there is not a sound spot in it. Simony has become so prevalent among the clergy that all secular and regular clerics, whether of high, middle or low rank, shamelessly buy and sell ecclesiastic livings without blame from anyone and much less with punishment. It looks as if our Lord had not driven the buyers and sellers from the Temple, but had rather invited them to remain there. Prebends, livings, dignities, rectorships, curacies, and altars are all for sale for money, or can be given in exchange for mistresses and concubines. They are staked at dice, lost and won. Even abbeys, priories, guardianships, professorships and readerships, and other posts, however insignificant they may be, are bought by ignorant, young, inexperienced, and stupid people, if only they possess money which they may have acquired by theft or in any other way."

No wonder that those organised terrible bands of robbers, the ill-famed companies, terrorised Italy, France, and all other European countries, mocked the Church, and displayed their atheism in the frankness of their cynical crimes. The German adventurer, Werner of Urslingen, who assumed the style of Duke of Guarineri and first assembled a large company from remnants of the bands he had broken up, a company which no one in Italy was capable of resisting, wore engraved on a medal attached to a chain round his neck the words, " Enemy of God, all charity, and mercy." The astonishing words which occur in the miracle play of Theophil prove that atheistic sentiments of this nature were by no means rare at this period : " O thou thoroughly wicked God, if I could but lay hands on Thee ! Truly I would tear Thee to pieces. I deny Thee, deny Thy faith and Thy power. I will go to the Orient, turn Mussulman, and live according to the law of Mahomet. He is a fool who puts his confidence in Thee ! "

The Luciferians, a sect of the fourteenth century, who were closely connected with the sect of the Brethren of the Free Mind and had many adherents among the mendicant orders, actually affirmed that God had obtained possession of heaven by usurpation, force, and injustice. When at church the faithful prayed, " Our Father which art in heaven," these heretics added when among themselves, " If He is in heaven it is only by force and injustice." The chief article of their Faith was that the unjust government of God over the world would some day be replaced by the rule of Lucifer, whom they worshipped with hymns and prayers.

In the companies in France which were recruited from the dregs of all nations, Spaniards, Englishmen, and Germans,

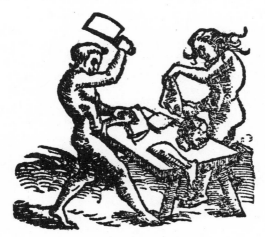

CANNIBALS FROM STARVATION.
From Lycosthenes.

were many runaway ecclesiasts, of whom the arch-priest Arnaud de Cervole was the most notorious. The conflicts between the nobility and the poor peasantry also led to the most horrible atrocities, by which the nickname Jacques Bonhomme, given to the peasants by the proud knights, has become coupled with deeds of incredible cruelty in the annals of history.

More than once it is reported that the raging peasant roasted noblemen in the presence of their wives and children, and then forced the wives to eat their flesh and ultimately murdered them after the most brutal violation. There can be no doubt that the Black Death contributed essentially to

the general deterioration of morals. In many places the
terrible famine which preceded and followed the plague led to
cannibalism. Children slaughtered their parents, parents their
children. The atrocities during the epidemics of plague in the
course of the Thirty Years' War represent the height of
European depravity. Of the numerous horrible stories one
only need be related as an example and which occurred at
Wollsin, a village a league and a half from Lippäen, in the
neighbourhood of Stettin, in the year 1638: "In the village
of Wollsin there was a man who hitherto had been honest
and pious and enjoyed a good reputation, his name was
Joachim Burghard. On account of the great famine, as for
some years he was unable to reap any harvest from his farms
and fields, he proceeded with two sons, Adam and Fritschen, to
the little town of Lippäen, telling his wife he was going to town
with the two boys to get his living; she should make her
preparations at home and follow them, as owing to the famine
they no longer had any means of preserving their lives. But
as they were so exhausted that their weakness prevented them
from reaching the town, and night came upon them too quickly,
they stopped at Kleinbroeden, which lies close to the road
where a brother of Joachim, Christoph Burghard, used to live,
but who had died of the plague together with his whole family,
with the exception of his sister's daughter, who had been
living with her cousins and who three days before had been
delivered of a son. He greeted the woman and congratulated
her on the child, and then with sorrow and weeping he related
his distress. But as according to the statement of the
youngest son, in the course of the last eleven weeks they had
eaten no bread or proper food, but only roots, and occasionally
acorns, which they had only consumed in the greatest necessity
as a means of sustaining life, their mental and physical constitution had undergone a change, and their human nature
had been converted into that of a wolf. Thus the above-
mentioned Burghard stepped up to the miserable bed on
which his niece, the daughter of his sister, was lying and
addressed her with savage words : ' Dear niece, have you
nothing for us to eat ? I and my sons must have something
to-day or we can no longer preserve life.' Whereupon the
woman, who had been lying in for six weeks, produced a key

and said he should look for himself, but he would find nothing
but a few boiled lettuce leaves. This had been her food from
the beginning of her lying in till her delivery. From the
moment that she lay down to the present she had had nothing
else to eat. When he now found that it was really so, he
agreed with his two sons to kill the sick woman and with her
flesh to stave off their hunger. He and his two sons set up
a horrible howl and bellow, and he said : 'Dear niece, pray to
God and implore mercy of Him, for now you must die and be
our food.' The sick woman was frightened, but could not
hope for help, but said : ' Dear uncle, you may eat me, but
not my child; I should be starved anyhow; God have mercy
on me ! ' Hereupon they set upon her with their knives,
stabbing her in the throat and the neck with great savagery
so that she should die soon, as she did without struggling or
screaming. They then cleaned the corpse and cut and scraped
the flesh from the bones, and, as they found a small vat containing rocksalt, they pickled a part of it, another part they
ate raw, and yet another slightly roasted, but most of it they
took back home, having abandoned their intention of going to
the town. When he reached home, Burghard said to his
wife : 'Dear wife, I am bringing you some meat; on my way
I found a pig, which I slaughtered, and of which I am now
bringing you a part. Perhaps it may be the means of preserving your life.' The woman, who was also starving, took
it greedily, boiled it a little, and ate it. But because the sick
woman was full of plague they all died within four days,
with the exception of the youngest son, Frederick Burghard,
who subsequently made a statement at Lippäen and died in
prison on the twelfth day. The gravediggers were ordered to
search the house and found more than half the flesh, which
was buried in the churchyard of the same place together with
the little child, who was found dead. And on the 2nd of June
the event was inscribed on a tablet and hung in the church
for everlasting memory."

In Italy, in the fourteenth century, during the plague,
there was neither " order nor justice and no one to administer
justice." In other countries things were much the same. So
soon as it came to the ears of the official or his commandant
that anyone was lying ill of the plague, Chrysopolitanus

relates of the epidemic at Parma in 1468, they immediately rushed to the house with a crowd of soldiers with great fury and din, and locked up the patient in the house or turned him out of the house; he then " had to make a journey to St. Leonard's, where the slaughter-house of the poor people was, and where there was much indecency and immorality. In this place terrible and inhuman cruelty and assassination flourished much more than love and friendship. In the town itself such disgraceful things were done and vices practised which no tongue could relate nor hand describe. The furious servants of the commandant went through the whole town and killed the pigs of the poor people and sold them." " As soon as the disease spread from the huts to the houses of the Patricians," Schoeppler reports on the conditions at Regensburg, " the whole body entrusted with the carrying out of the plague regulations fled and left the execution of their *most urgent orders* to a plague steward. He, a bankrupt merchant or a notorious adulterer or some other man of doubtful honesty, who in normal times occupied the post of prison master at some institution for the improvement of vicious men and women now used as plague hospital, entrusted the execution of his duties to his rough servants, who were drawn from the dregs of the people and who under pretence of combating the plague practised all the arts of hell on the defenceless patients —women, children, and corpses."

Everywhere the gravediggers and nurses were taken from the dregs of the population—they were largely liberated galley-slaves, as no one else would undertake so dangerous a service. " Only on the galleys are people to be found who are so weary of themselves and their lives that they are not terrified by any danger. Life is indifferent to them ; when once relieved of their chains they delight in their new profession in which they are fed, clothed, and lodged as they have never been before in their lives. It is most important to preserve the life of a criminal if he is to sacrifice it in the service of those attacked by the plague " (Antrechau).

The gravediggers were called " Becchini " or " Monatti." The latter designation is said to be derived from the solitude in which they were obliged to live, as no one was allowed to speak to them. In Toulon they were called ravens; in Russia, where they were more dreadful than plague and death, they were known as Mortus.

The most impressive description of the atrocities committed by the Monatti is to be found in Manzoni's "Betrothed." An examination of the sources of this description, which makes our hair stand on end, proves that Manzoni remained far behind reality. Let us hear the celebrated French surgeon, Ambroise Paré, on the conditions in Paris : " The worst of all is that the rich, the higher town officials and all persons vested with official authority, flee among the first at the outbreak of the plague, so that administration of justice is rendered impossible and no one can obtain his rights. General anarchy and confusion then set in and that is the worst evil by which the commonwealth can be assailed ; for that is the moment when the dissolute bring another and still worse plague into the town. They penetrate into the houses, rob and plunder to their hearts' content, and frequently cut the throats of the sick. In the town of Paris people have been found who with the help of these worthy elements would inform their enemy that he is suffering from the plague, although there was nothing the matter with him. And on the day when he should have appeared in the law court they had him seized by these villains and carried to the hospital by force. How could he, an isolated individual, offer resistance against a crowd. If on the way he appealed for the assistance and pity of the people in the streets, the murderers prevented him and shouted louder than he, so that no one could understand him ; or they maintained that the disease had rendered him delirious. By such means they succeeded in driving him to the hospital, where he was locked up with those suffering from the plague. A few days after he would die from despair or in consequence of the infection, his death having been previously paid for in hard cash."

But, without being bribed, the Monatti penetrated into the houses of the healthy, and dragged husbands, wives, and children to the plague hospital if they were refused money. The business was so lucrative that young men of the criminal class took to it. They fastened bells to their feet and moved about the streets as if they were Monatti, vested with public authority, penetrated into the houses, robbed, violated, and blackmailed to their hearts' content. At Milan it happened on several occasions that such pretended and real gravediggers met in the same house and engaged in bloody conflicts.

All chroniclers relate of the callous and repugnant manner in which corpses were treated. It was terrible for the survivors to see the Monatti dragging the corpses of the dead along the ground, fearful to hear no other bells than those worn by these monsters on their legs. From all countries it is reported that the gravediggers threw infected matter from their carts so as to stimulate the epidemic which for them was a time of luxury. Their spite was particularly directed against the rich, who suffered less from the epidemic. The people, who largely believed that the disease was artificially produced by the rich, assisted them in their criminal behaviour and approved of their maxim that the rich should die as well as the poor.

The violation of female corpses was the order of the day, and it happened that women in a comatose state, recovering consciousness at the moment of violation, were actually killed by terror. In Vienna many of the plague workers who had been as serving nurses had to be arrested, as they had rendered more than three hundred women pregnant.

Daniel Defoe relates that watchmen who were appointed to guard the locked-up houses broke into them and hurled corpses still warm into the corpse cart. Even at the beginning of the eighteenth century it still occurred that the attendants, " to help the patients to get over it more quickly, placed a piece of a death's head (skull) under their pillow ; squeezed the noses of those too weak to resist, under pretence of absorbing the poison ; placed moist bread in their mouths or simply turned the very weak upon their faces ; all these abominable crimes were, according to Saxon laws, punishable by execution with the sword or on the wheel."

From the Mark Brandenburg it is reported that during long epidemics people, having grown tired of constant burying, did not only take the dead to the burying trenches, but also the living who had lost all strength, more from starvation than from the plague, and threw the living and the dead together into the graves so as to save the trouble of frequent journeys, leaving them to perish there or even burying them alive, although many might have recovered. In Thorn in 1580 a blind attendant at the hospital of St. George was tortured with burning tongs, and then drawn and quartered for having strangled forty people and violated two maidens of tender age.

At Vienna on the 1st December, 1679, the Master of the Lazaretto was hanged at the gate of his hospital because, in addition to other frauds, he had entered 246 patients too many in his books. The memorial tablet on his grave, which is written in Latin, terminates with the following verse in German :

> Here lies buried in this grave
> A man who stole like any knave,
> And though the plague his life did spare,
> The hangman claimed him as his share,
> Of our plague house he was the head,
> And yet he stole the children's bread.

A case reported from Regensburg is particularly typical : " A street-sweeper of the name of Zacherl was appointed gravedigger at the pest-house ; he was at constant logger-heads with the cook. When the latter died of the plague he laid her over his shoulder and carried her to the plague burying ground; he stripped her naked of her clothes and, as he only found one single small coin on her, he tore a strip from her chemise, rolled it up like a sausage and inserted it in her uterus, the coin he thrust into her nostril and, hurling her into the trench, he said : ' Lie there, you beast; you never would cook me a good soup.' "

" At Magdeburg during the plague epidemic of 1625 a maid, who had been sent by her master to fetch beer, encountered in the house where she was to fetch it a company of gravediggers and plague attendants, one of whom seized her and forced her to dance with him. At the end of the dance he threw his cloak over her head, breathed in her face and said in a rough voice : ' Ha, wench, that will do for you ; you'll have to pay for it.' The maid was so terrified that she fell ill as soon as she returned home and died the night after."

The dread of the pest-houses to which at the outbreak of an epidemic not only those who had contracted disease but also the healthy inhabitants of the house were brought was terrible. Wherever possible cases of plague were kept secret and the dead disposed of quietly ; they were buried in the cellar or under the boards of the floor. Fear of the depraved behaviour of the hospital attendants was at Milan so great, particularly among the women, that many committed suicide rather than be taken to the pest-house. The number of suicides increased so alarmingly that the officials threatened to exhibit publicly the corpses of all who had destroyed themselves. This threat proved efficacious.

Even during the last plague at Marseilles the hospitals were described as the ante-room of death. A poem of this time gives a lively description : " God preserve you from headache. If you have it, make clear to yourself you are done ; it is time to think of your end. You are taken to chapel. A priest eagerly orders you to confess. Think of your bygone misdeeds, for already your agony is upon you. Let us evoke together the Virgin Mary. They recite to you prayers for the dying. The blood refuses to flow in your body. You must tread the same path as those who died before you have trodden. Your heart is wrung with pain, for you hear nothing but sighs, cries of terror, and the sad wail of the dreaming and of those raving in their fever. Alas! good God, I dare not continue. I feel that grief will render me unconscious. When dawn breaks you hear the sick attendant come and say : ' Lift up your shirts.' When the surgeons come they will examine your boils. You are all drawn up in a row when they arrive. They look at you, and in their hands they bear plasters and instruments. They pass you like a gust of wind. What cries, what moans. Not for a moment is there peace. You hear nothing but cries of pain. One says : ' Oh, how my boils burn.' Another : ' The pain in my thigh is intolerable.' A third : ' I have pains higher up.' Others remain motionless in their place. Now you see the corpse-bearers coming, and that is an evil sign. Roughly they seize the corpses by the head or by the legs, and cruelly drag them through the ward. They are capable of striking you dead. To see all that is heart-rending. A few minutes later and they will be bearing you to the grave, and you will be shovelled in without ceremony, like a dead ass is thrown upon the field."

How callous the healthy were towards the sick outside the

pest-houses is also shown by a description of the plague at Marseilles. No one rendered assistance. If they were thirsty they had to moisten their tongues in the gutter like cattle. They were driven away from benches and walls, and house-owners poured out water in front of their houses or scattered the lees of wine to keep them away.

An example quoted by Sahm in his " History of the Plague in East Prussia " shows to what madness the dread of the plague occasionally gave rise. The steward of the estate, Peisten, had a half-witted old woman, who had been nursing plague patients in the neighbourhood, placed alive in a coffin, and made the local gendarme fire at the coffin till she expired.

We have already heard from Luther of the malicious manner in which plague patients infected healthy people : Nicolas Selneccerus also relates similar cases : " Thus godless, desperate arch-rogues and villains are to be found who, when God has stricken them with this plague in their bodies, go to churches, markets, and houses for the sole purpose of infecting and poisoning others, and thus, as they believe, getting rid of their disease, or simply because they don't want to have the plague alone. I know of a case in which a man who visited another, and blew and breathed into his face, afterwards confessed that he had done so to get rid of his disease by passing it on."

In Normandy sorcerers particularly advised patients to pass on their plague. A case is reported from the time of the epidemic at Danzic in which a man fastened to the peep-hole of his neighbour, with whom he was on bad terms, a plaster covered with pus which had been on a plague boil. When he thrust out his head to see who was there it stuck to his beard without his noticing it, and for some time he went about with it, till his wife saw it and asked him what he had on his beard ? Upon which they were both seized with great terror.

To what excesses hate may lead among scholars is shown by a case reported by Arnim : " A Greek manuscript had carried the infection of the plague to the celebrated Hemken-gripper at Leyden, who in his malicious joy of refuting his learned adversary Zahnebrecker had neglected every pre-caution. The manuscript arrived on a ship infected by the

plague and should have been passed through vinegar.
Hemkengripper's servant recognised the disease as soon as
her master was attacked.   But the latter ordered her to keep
silent. He sent a ceremonial offer of reconciliation to
Zahnebrecker, who, in accordance with his frank character,
immediately accepted. At a feast in honour of the reconciliation Hemkengripper embraced him, and infected him so
effectually with his first kiss of reconciliation that both died
nearly within an hour.   Half the town followed them first as
mourners to the grave and then as corpses to their own graves,
and only few suspected that their whole misfortune was due
to the hatred of two scholars."

It was in a lesser degree due to atrocities of this nature
which, after all, were only of sporadic occurrence, than to
the incapacity to believe that so uncanny a disease as the
plague could be attributable to natural causes, that the fateful
misconception of the artificial production of the plague
developed.   Already in Livy we find the belief that human
malice is capable of artificially producing an epidemic among
human beings and animals. He relates that under the con-
sulate of M. Claudius Marcellus and C. Halelius one hundred
and seventy persons were arrested for strewing powders
productive of disease and were put to death. Seneca also
believed that wells were poisoned and that pestilence could
be artificially produced. Moses and Aaron "took ashes of the
furnace and stood before Pharaoh ; and Moses sprinkled it
up toward heaven, and it became a boil breaking forth with
blains upon men and upon beast " (Exod. ix. 10).

Archbishop Agobardus relates that the great cattle epidemic
in the year 800 was produced artificially by Grimvaldus,
Duke of Benevento. Prompted by enmity for Emperor
Charlemagne, he sent people to France, who strewed poison
over the fields, mountains, and meadows. Several of the
miscreants were caught and put to death. The marvellous
part of the matter was that none of those who, under torture,
confessed their crime was capable of explaining how such an
efficacious and secret powder could be prepared that was
noxious to cattle alone and to practically no other animal.
On a broadsheet printed at Prague in 1682 we find information relating to an epidemic among cattle produced by

witchcraft. The conclusion of this broadsheet runs : "It is reported that in Switzerland, close to Lindau, there were two sorcerers who achieved the following : Two Frenchmen in Switzerland went to a woman who was lying in and demanded three drops of her milk and three hairs from her head, which she refused them, but told them to come back in two hours ; her husband was not at home—before the two hours had passed he returned. Then the woman told him what the two persons had demanded from her. Her husband ordered her to take three drops of cow's milk and three hairs from the tail of a foal, and when they came back to give them to them. And behold the two persons came back at the time appointed, and demanded the same things as before ; the woman gave them to them, as her husband had ordered ; they took them and went away with them. And, as one subsequently confessed, they put them together in a glass and used them for the purpose of sorcery. They proceeded in the following manner : They made a boy climb up a tree with the glass and told him he should look into the glass. They asked him a first and a second time what he saw in the glass ? He replied: 'Nothing.' But when they asked him a third time, he replied that he saw a whole field full of dead cattle. When they heard this they cried, 'We have been cheated.' Shortly after, these two miscreants were to be arrested, but one immediately sprang into the water and drowned himself. The other was caught and was subsequently immured alive, but before he was asked if there was no way of saving the cattle. Whereupon he replied : Yes, there would develop on the tongue of the cattle a small boil. This should be opened with a fine silver lancet till the raw flesh was laid bare, then honey should be rubbed on it. But this sorcery was not intended for the cattle but for human beings ; for if the woman had given them some of her milk and her hair the epidemic would have come over human beings, that was why they had said, 'We have been cheated.' The Lindau beadle stated that he himself had been close to the wall when the man was immured, and that the sorcerer had said that this epidemic would spread every two days a distance that could be covered in a walk of two hours. The cattle would suffer sixteen hours before falling dead. If help were not forthcoming in the first eight hours nothing would be of avail. And all this proved to be correct."

In reply to the question how it was possible that an artificially produced plague could have such virulence and strength and carry off more people than a natural plague, we receive the genuinely mediæval reply : because to Satan all poisonous animals, herbs, and minerals are known throughout, and he is thus easily able to extract a quintessence from them. The pestilential poison was mostly enclosed in ointment by the sorcerers, and could thus be transported through towns and whole empires. Certainly many of the abstruse brains of the Middle Ages have endeavoured to prepare such ointments, and were themselves convinced of the efficacy of their preparations. Even such scholars as Athanasius Kircher and Antoninus Portus pretend to have been conversant with the art, but were wisely silent about it. " The composition of plague ointment and plague powder I will pass over in silence and not bring this work of the lower world again to the light of day " (Kircher). Quercetanus relates that Swiss people confessed to him and his colleagues that they obtained instruction in the preparation of plague poisons and antidotes from the Devil. The plague poison was composed mainly of aconite, arsenic, and napellum mixed with other poisons, which he also refuses to mention. Paracelsus also narrates that in his time the plague was artificially produced at Rothweil, Wasserberg, Passau, Eger, St. Veit, Willach, etc., by the burying of diabolical mummies (see page 95). Many plague regulations had special paragraphs referring to ointment spreaders and greasers, as they were called. Thus in the Venetian plague regulations for the years 1576 to 1577 the twenty-second regulation runs : "Anyone who within forty days from the publication of these regulations can denounce any member of the company engaged in greasing with poisonous ointments doors, handles and bolts, or other things, shall receive a reward of 500 crowns and shall be granted permission to kill two bandits."

Particular terror was caused by a band of 500 miscreants who at Genoa, Leghorn, and Lucca, as well as in Neapolitan territory and in the Abruzzi, were said to have smeared walls, windows, doorposts, trapdoors in the houses, canals, wells, church pews, and holy water containers with poisonous matter, in order to produce a general epidemic. Although a close look-out was kept for these poisoners and 2,000 crowns' reward was offered to anyone who lead to their discovery, " not a single one could be found." Everywhere, in all countries, it was believed that the traces of such miscreants were to be seen, and thus the general hallucination became coupled with the most terrible ideas of persecution. " No longer did one neighbour trust another—husbands and wives, parents and children, brothers and sisters, all suspected one another." After the Reformation it was commonly assumed that Germany was the home of the plague-makers, and in Naples and Milan plague-making was attributed to the Lutherans. Several authors praise King Philip IV because he caused all the Spanish coasts to be carefully guarded so that the raging madness of Lutherism should not be introduced into the country by stealth.

In Rostock, a Catholic ecclesiastic, Hildensem, who had been tending the sick and dying, was suspected of plague-making. He was said to have been bribed with Jewish money. He was cast into a narrow prison where, with fettered limbs and gagged mouth, he lay for twenty-six weeks on bread and water. During the cold of winter his feet were for some time roasted in the fire, and he was tortured in other ways. When, subsequently, he was found innocent, he was made to swear an oath to retain silence on what had been done to him and not to raise any complaints.

During the plague at Lyons in 1564 " the heretics, when they saw the number of their adherents decreasing, had recourse to the children of Satan. With ointment received from hell they smeared the houses of the Catholics. But by the grace of God it was achieved that the plague recoiled on the heretics and that most deaths were among the sectarians. During the plague in Spain in 1630 it was averred that it was the heretics from Geneva who had invented a diabolical poisonous powder to kill the people. In consequence of this all Frenchmen, as if they had all been from Geneva, became so unpopular that at Madrid names were called after them in the streets and they were exposed to all kinds of insults. Ultimately a royal edict was issued that all Frenchmen in

Spain had to be registered. This edict had the following terrible introduction : "As some enemies of humanity who, as rebels against the Catholic religion, have determined the destruction of the human race and have invented a powder by the spreading of which they have produced the plague in the territory of Milan and other royal territories, anyone who can denounce a person engaged in such works shall be rewarded with 20,000 ducats."

The most celebrated plague-makers' trial was that of Milan. At last it was believed that the traces of a great conspiracy of poisoners had been discovered. On the rack, which at that time no one considered unjust or barbaric, the barber John Jacob Mora and the Public Commissioner of the Office of Health, William Platea, as well as some other unfortunate individuals, had confessed what the judges and the exceedingly excited people wished to hear. As their chief they denounced Don Juan Gaetano de Padilla, the son of the Spanish commandant of the fortress, who, while suffering from syphilis, had unfortunately had recourse to the services of the barber. On the 17th July they were executed in the following manner :

"First they were placed upon a cart and driven to the place of execution. On the way they were pinched with glowing tongs at every place where poison had been smeared ; before Mora's house they both had their right hands cut off and subsequently they were both broken on the wheel, being placed living on the wheel and strangled after six hours, their corpses were burnt with fire, their ashes strewn upon the water, Mora's dwelling was pulled down and in its place a column of disgrace was erected with the following inscription : 'On this spot stood the barber's shop of John Jacob Mora who conspired, together with William Platea, an official of the public health offices during an epidemic of plague, by smearing mortal ointments to contrive the cruel death of many.' Both were condemned as guilty of high treason to be pinched with glowing tongs on high wagons, and after having had their right hands cut off, to be placed on the wheel, there to remain for six hours and finally to be burnt. And that nothing should remain of such criminals the Senate decreed that their possessions should be confiscated and their ashes strewn in the river. For the everlasting memory of their misdeed it was further decreed that the scene of their crime should be levelled to the ground and never reconstructed, and in its stead a column should be erected which should be called the 'column of disgrace.' All good citizens keep away from the place, so that the unhappy ground may not defile you. Dated the 1st day of August 1630. The President of the Public Health Council, Marc Anton Monti ; the President of the High Council, John Baptist Trotto ; the Representative of the Royal Justice, John Baptist Visconti."

The Devil, at whose suggestion the two unfortunate men are said to have prepared the poison, was seen by all people at the outbreak of the epidemic. He appeared in the form of a prince in most costly attire with a suite of many servants driving about at noon in an open coach. He was said to have the appearance of a man of about fifty who had already turned grey. He said his name was Prince Mammon. He also went to many who had contracted the plague and asked if they desired to be healed. Some who expressed the wish he immediately restored ; others who refused his services he finished off with many blows. One of those who pretended to have conversed with him related the following :

One day when he was standing in the Piazza del Duomo he saw a coach drive up, it was drawn by six white horses and in it, accompanied by a large suite, a man of terrifying appearance was to be seen. His brow was lowering, his eyes agleam, his hair matted, his lips menacing and imperious. While open-mouthed he stood staring at this curious apparition, the coachman pulled the reins and stopped the coach and the prince invited him to get in and have a drive with him. From politeness he accepted and he was driven about the town until at last they stopped at the gate of a certain house which he entered together with the stranger. This house, the narrator continues, was very like the man who had invited him to get into the coach and whose orders were obeyed implicitly by all in the house. The description of the house shows a remarkable similarity with Homer's description of Circe's cave. The terrible and majestic, the charming and the horrible were standing cheek by jowl. Here light and the sheen of precious stones, there darkness and artificial night. Uncanny forms were grouped in a circle, broad wastes,

woods and gardens were scattered around, and to the screech
of vultures water rushed with resounding din into huge recep-
tacles.   The narrator maintains further that he was shown in
the house immense treasures, chests filled with gold and
precious stones, and he was promised as much of them as he
desired if he would swear by the name of the prince to lend
a helping hand in all that was required from him.   If he was
willing to accept, the sign of consent should be that he should
walk round the prince with upraised finger and strike the
ground with his knuckle.   When he manfully refused to do
this he suddenly found himself transferred to the Piazza del
Duomo, where he had entered the coach.   When one reads this
fantastic yarn, which was circulated in Germany particularly
by broadsheets at the present day, and considers how few
centuries it lies behind us, it seems nearly incredible.   In
later years the protest was discovered which Mora and Platea
had dictated to their confessor on the night preceding the
execution of their sentence :   " In the name of Jesus, the
31st of July 1630.   I, Jacobus Mora, barber, enter protest
against my sentence to death and, as I do not wish to leave
this world with a weight upon my conscience, I once more
protest and declare in this document that all who in the
course of the trial were accused by me to have been concerned
in the manipulation of pestilential ointments are completely
innocent.   I write this in the presence of the Capuchin fathers
and witnesses for the salvation of my soul."

It is to be assumed that among the gravediggers there
were really men who spread poison.   It is reported from
Leyden that they defiled the walls with plague pus to drive
the inhabitants from the houses so that they might acquire
all that was left behind.   In Leipzig several people are said
to have made use of the services of poisoners and sorcerers to
get rid of their relations and reap legacies.   It is also credible
that thieves, and foremost among them the gravediggers,
circulated alarming rumours of this nature so that the people
should leave their houses and make it easy for them to steal.
In any case, the imagination of the people was terribly excited
and highly strung and, as they attributed the disease rather
to magic than to natural causes, they demanded victims and
could only be appeased by the ruthless execution of the

pretended miscreants. Full of horror, they heard the confessions of the plague smearers, which for the most part originated on the rack. One of them confessed that when smearing his ointments, he felt the same pleasure as the sportsman when he shoots birds for fun, being unable to obtain any better game. Another maintained that for him there could be no human pleasure which could equal it. In many places it was asserted that the plague immediately decreased if the heads

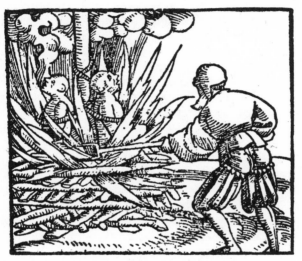

BURNING OF PLAGUE SPREADERS.
From Sebastian Muenster's " Cosmographie."

were cut off the bodies of witches and sorcerers who had already been buried. Mohsen reports that in German districts where there were no Jews, in Saxony at Leipzig, Plauen, Weyda, and Wolkenstein, as well as in the Archbishopric of Magdeburg and in various towns of Silesia such as Brieg, Guhrau, Reichenstein, Frankenstein, and Praussnitz, the gravediggers were collected from all parishes, forced to confess by means of torture and legally condemned to be burnt alive publicly. On the 10th of September 1606, there were arrested at Frankenstein, on confession, two gravedigger assistants who were under the influence of drink, two master gravediggers,

Wenzel Foerster who had been a gravedigger for about twenty-eight years, and Freidiger of Striegau ; on the 14th of September the wives of the two masters, together with Caspar Schleiniger, gravedigger and corpse-bearer at Frankenstein ; and on the 18th of September old Caspar Schetts, a messenger and beggar aged eighty-seven years, on a charge of strewing poison during the plague; on the 4th of October Susanna Matz, the daughter of the late municipal official, together with her mother Magdalena on a charge of strewing posion, etc.

On September 12, 1607, there was found at Wenzel Foerster's, the old gravedigger's house, one year after his execution, a whole chest full of paper bags with poison powder by which the plague was to be spread. On the 15th of October, a gravedigger Johann Laken and his son, a boy of fourteen years, were beheaded and their heads and bodies burnt on a wood pile. Together with these, seventeen persons who had strewn and prepared powders were sentenced and burnt.

In Guhrau, on their confession, the gravediggers were flayed and their bodies pinched with red hot tongs. Criminal proceedings on charges of creating plague may be traced till the end of the seventeenth century. Roch's chronicle of calamities is full of them, and the examples quoted from it prove that not only gravediggers but also other people, particularly vagabonds and vagrants, were pinched with tongs and burnt for strewing poison powders.

CHAPTER VIII

PERSECUTION OF THE JEWS

The secret heads of the Jewish community at Toledo—Jewish spells—The burning of lepers—The first pogroms—Legal massacres and profitable confiscations—Papal bull against the persecution of the Jews—Anti-Jewish guilds—Anti-Jewish princes—The adventures of the mystic Suso—Privileged usury of the Jews—Fantastic rate of interest—Jew baiting and the Church—Pretended ritual murders—Jewish tenacity—Superiority of the Jewish physicians—A saying of Jean Paul—The fable of the three rings.

Appendices : A letter from the municipality of Cologne—The well poisoning trial at Chillon, 1348—Complaint of Jews of neglect by Christian physicians—A testament.

It is only the systematic extermination of the Jews which reveals the whole confusion and irresponsibility of these dark ages. If I first treated the persecution of the Christian grave-diggers and sorcerers, I did so in the endeavour to tone down the impression of horror. The massacres of the Jews in the fourteenth century are so deeply revolting, because the ruling classes, so well as the clergy and the educated classes of that time, were perfectly conscious of the lack of foundation in the accusations brought by the people against the Jews; but from fear of the rabble and still more for the sake of material profit, not only held their peace, but in the most cruel manner participated in the slaughter of the innocent victims. It is impossible to ascertain by whom the terrible assertion that the Black Death was artificially produced by the Jews was first made. It must be assumed that the rumour originated in many places at the same time.

As pope and emperor had come to loggerheads, as one of the innumerable versions expressed it, the Jews were of the opinion that the destruction of the Christians had been decreed. And therefore they had secretly conspired to exterminate them by poison. The specific order to poison the wells was said to have been issued by the secret heads of the community at Toledo, who had procured the poison for the Black Death from the Orient or had prepared it themselves from spiders, owls, and other poisonous animals. Orders for the forging of the currency, the murder of Christian children, etc., were said to have emanated from the same quarter. Others maintained that the plague had been produced by Jewish spells. The old myth of the poisoning of wells was first revived in the South of France, and from there spread over the whole of Europe. But at first there was no agreement as to whom this terrible crime was to be attributed. The nobility suspected the common people, the hatred of the poor caused them to charge the rich. Many considered the Jews the perpetrators of this godless outrage, others again the lepers. Already in 1313 all lepers in France had been burnt without reason by order of Philip the Fair. For the suspicion that they had poisoned the wells was simply trumped up to cover the fear of being infected by them. Ultimately it was agreed that the Jews were the well-poisoners, and as early as May 1348 in a town in Provence all Jewish inhabitants fell victims to the rage of the populace. The burning of Jews was particularly thorough at Narbonne and Carcassone. In Burgundy alone fifty thousand Jews were massacred in the most cruel manner. Although the Pope in the two bulls of July 4th and September 26th, 1348, forbade the plundering and slaughtering of Jews on pain of excommunication, the accusation passed like wildfire through Savoy and Burgundy. In September 1348 the rack tore a confession from the Jews on the shores of the lake of Geneva. Already on September 21 a solemn resolution was passed at Zurich never again to admit Jews into the town. The Council of the little town of Zofingen in Argau forwarded little bags of poison, alleged to have been found in the cisterns, to the authorities of the towns on the upper Rhine. And from Berne solemn exhortations were addressed to the towns of Basle, Freiburg in Breisgau and Strasbourg to prosecute the Jews as poisoners. At Benne-feld in Alsace, a formal diet was held at which bishops, lords and barons, as well as representatives of the counts and municipalities, discussed what measures were to be taken against the Jews. The deputies of the town of Strasbourg

raised their voice in defence of the persecuted. But, as the
Bishop of Strasbourg proved himself a violent fanatic, they
aroused loud dissention and were assailed with questions as to
why they had covered in their wells and removed their buckets.
It was thus that a bloody resolution was carried and at the
hands of the rabble, willing to obey the summons of the great
and high clergy, found but too willing executors. As in all
cases the rack here again provided detailed confessions. One
of those subjected to it asserted that all the Jews in the neighbourhood of the Lake of Geneva had held a formal council
outside the gates of Villeneuf to discuss by what means they
could best poison the Christians. From another the confession was torn that at Venice, in Apulia, Calabria, and at
Toulouse he had thrown little bags of poison into the wells.

The Strasbourg chronicle of Michael Kleinlawel reports in
1348 :

> And at that time, when death did rage
> In countries far and near,
> Yea, and throughout all Christenage,
> Of this it seemed quite clear,
> The Jews were guilty of this crime
> As all around was said,
> By poisoning wells at this same time,
> As on the rack when laid,
> Some (as were stated) to have done
> Themselves confessed it true,
> And, therefore, without mercy shown
> Were burnt in many a lieu.
> And death in this dread form
> To Strasbourg now drew nigh,
> And of its people killed a swarm
> Young, old and low and high.
> Particularly in forty-nine,
> When sixteen thousand died,
> The citizens did much incline
> To measures elsewhere tried.
> Three masters stoutly did resist
> All measures of this kind,
> The Jews they wanted to assist
> And loudly spake their mind.
> The people to the minster trooped,
> The masters soon must yield,
> And on the Jews they quickly swooped,
> Revenge to seek afield.

With bitter cries they soon were caught,
Wherever they might be,
And on one day were burnt to naught
Two hundred or near by.

One Sabbath the sorrowful procession of the victims destined to death moved, surrounded by the raging rabble, towards the Jewish cemetery, where a huge common grave was prepared for them on the flaming pile. On their way to execution the inhuman crowd had even torn their clothes from their backs, and in their greed gloated over the quantity of money found sewn in them. But few Jews, who had consented to be baptised, several women conspicuous by their beauty, and many children, who were received in the Christian community, escaped the tragic fate of their co-religionists.

A resolution of the municipal council decreed that for the course of a whole century no Jews should be allowed to settle at Strasbourg. All pledges and bonds the council ordered to be returned to the debtors and all money found to be distributed among the artisans. Many, however, refused to accept such filthy blood money, but on the advice of their confessors made it over to the monasteries; they were horrified at the scenes of murderous greed over which the enraged populace seemed to have forgotten the plague.

It was believed to be a good work if churches were repaired with bricks and stones taken from the burnt houses and destroyed graves of the Jews and new belfries erected. At Muehlhausen all the Jews were slaughtered, at Nordhausen at least a part of them. The Landgrave Frederick of Thuringia-Meisen, an ardent enemy of the Jews, was so annoyed that in the latter town not all had been exterminated that in May he addressed an urgent exhortation to the municipal council of Nordhausen to burn all Jews immediately " for the praise and honour of God and the benefit of Christianity." At Basle, the town council was impelled, by the threatening attitude of the guilds, who with unfurled banners marched to the Town Hall, to burn the Jews and prohibit their settling in the town for two hundred years. The diabolical scheme was then conceived of imprisoning all Jews in a wooden shed on an island in the Rhine, outside the town, and then setting the shed on fire. As the chronicler reports these atrocities were perpetrated exclusively on the tempestuous urging of the populace and without legal sanction. Schaffhausen formed a laudable exception and protected the local Jews. The inhabitants of Mayence made such fires for the burning of their Jews—to the number of twelve thousand—that the lead in the window-panes and the bells of St. Quirius church were melted. A part of the Jews of Speyer were massacred by a raving crowd and their bodies, placed in empty wine-barrels, allowed to drift down the Rhine. Despair, however, inspired the majority with the heroic courage to escape from the hands of the fiendish rabble by setting fire to their own houses and perishing in the flames. It is related of a Jew of Constance, who had been baptised to save himself, that he repented having renounced the faith of his forefathers and set fire to his house, burning himself and all the inmates of the house, together with his precious stones and valuables. While the fire was raging he shouted through the window to the crowd below that they would not live as Christians, but rather die as pious Jews. At Esslingen the whole Jewish congregation were burnt in their synagogue, which they themselves had set on fire ; and in other towns mothers were seen to throw their children on the burning pile rather than to permit of their being baptised, and then fling themselves into the flames after them. On July 24, 1349, the Jews were burnt at Frankfort. Here again, as at Oppenheim, many escaped from the hands of their executioners by burning themselves. At Nuremberg all the Jews were murdered, and at Eger the gloomy " Murder Alley " still bears testimony to the massacre of the Jews in 1350. In the Thuringian towns Gotha, Eisenach, Dennerstaedt, Kreuzburg, Arnstadt, Ilmen, Nebra, Wiehe, Herbsleben, Thomasbruecken, Frankenhausen, and Weissensee the Jews were slaughtered to the last man. The council of the town of Erfurt was anxious to save the Jews, and would have stayed the hands of the burghers; but in spite of this more than a hundred were slaughtered, the rest, about three thousand, set fire to their houses and burnt themselves together with their families.

In the North of Germany, where only a few Jews were settled, the appearance of the great plague in 1350 was the first cause of their persecution. As is reported by the

Brunswick town secretary the Jew Rumbold carried on his
nefarious handicraft in Prussia from Easter to the day of
St. Gallus, 1350, and poisoned many people. At Elbing alone
more than nine thousand perished in consequence from St.
Bartholomew's to Christmas. In the same manner numerous
inhabitants were said to have been killed at Koenigsberg,
Marienburg, Preussisch, Holland Heiligenbeil, Frauenburg, and
Muehlhausen by poison. In the Hanse towns, Wismar, Rostock,
Stralsund, and Greifswald, the few Jews settled there were

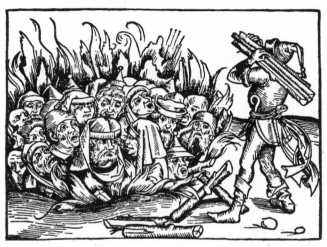

BURNING OF THE JEWS.
From Schedel's Chronicle.

partially burnt, partially immured alive. Where there were
no adherents of the Mosaic faith, as, for instance, in the territory to the Teutonic knights, the converted Jews were hunted
down and burnt at the stake. In July 1350 the councillors
of Luebeck informed Duke Otto of Brunswick-Lueneburg that
they, as well as the councillors of Stralsund, Rostock, Wismar,
and Wisby, had apprehended some miscreants on the island
of Gothland, and that these confessed that they had been
hired by some Jews, whose names they stated, to poison
Christians. A circumstantial confession had been made by a
certain Dietrich, who had been burnt on July 1, 1350, on

Gothland. Before his death this man confessed in the presence of the assembly of the people that, in the town of Dussel, he had received from a Jew called Aaron, the son of the rich Jew Salomon at Hanover, thirty marks and three hundred little bags of poison, and with these had poisoned the wells at Hanover, Hildesheim, and other towns of Lower Saxony. When there the great plague broke out, he fled to Luebeck, and on his way there lost the thirty marks at dice. At Luebeck a Jew called Moisen came to him at his inn and handed him ten marks and a box of poison, with which he embarked for Frauenburg on the Prussian coast, where, as well as at Memel and other places, he continued his poisonous activity. Finally the council of Luebeck conjured the Duke of Lueneburg to exterminate the Jews in his territory, for it was to be feared that the ravages of the plague among the Christians would never end so long as the Jews found protection with the princes.

In Austria the chief persecutions of the Jews were at Krems, Stein, and Mautern. A crowd of people from the neighbourhood collected and advanced to Krems. The first Jews who encountered the crowd were murdered, their houses were entered, plundered and destroyed. The few who at the first approach of the rabble took refuge in the citadel were fortunate. The commandant Meissau granted them protection ; they were the only ones who escaped the general slaughter. The others to escape the barbarities of the rabble set fire to their own houses and perished in the flames. Duke Albrecht sent a company of men-at-arms against the raging people and had their leaders arrested. Three were hanged, some died in prison, and others purchased their release. The town of Mautern was mulcted six hundred pounds, and the towns Krems and Stein four hundred pounds. Mild as the punishment was in proportion to the crime, it was greatly resented as unjust, and Albrecht was upbraided as a friend of the heretic Jews. The Count of the Palatinate of the Rhine, Ruprecht, also made himself hated by his protection of the Jews. It was said that he had been bribed by the Jews, and the people wanted to wreak vengeance on him as on all " Jew princes."

In Italy and in Spain the Jews fared no better. They found refuge only in Lithuania, where Duke Bodeslav of

Poland (1227-79) had already granted them religious liberty,
and particularly in Poland where King Casimir the Great, at the
request of his Jewish mistress Esther, gave them protection—
a fact which explains the large number of Jews in Poland at
the present time.   In England the Jews were in some places
accused of spreading the plague, but were not persecuted.

How deeply rooted the belief in the poisoning of wells was
among the people is shown by the circumstance that not only
Jews but in many places also Christians fell victim to this
fixed idea.   How easily anyone might be accused is best shown
by the story related by the South German mystic Suso [1] in
his autobiography.

In 1348 he had been sent on business by the convent of
his Constance monastery to Alsatia.   A half-witted, and at
the same time malicious, lay-brother accompanied him on his
journey.   This man had mingled with the crowd at an Alsatian
fair, consisting of pilgrims, pedlars and soldiers, and in this
company got drunk, while Suso, with his mailbag over his
shoulder, was attending to his ecclesiastic business.   By his
foolish talk the lay-brother roused the suspicion that he
might be one of the prowling poison spreaders.   In consequence
of this he was finally arrested and taken to the tower to be
examined.   To get himself out of the scrape, the rogue declared
that not he but Suso, who was momentarily absent, had been
instructed to poison the wells and had the poison bags in his
possession.   That was the reason why Suso had set out early
in the morning, probably he had gone to the village well,
whereas he himself had spent the livelong day drinking at
the inn.   Immediately the rabble set out to look for the
absent man with loud shouts.   With sword, spear, and halbert
they marched through the village, breaking into houses and
huts, searching beds and straw mattresses, everywhere they
believed he was hidden.   With no suspicion of this incident,
Suso had in the meantime returned to his inn, where he heard
the stupid story.   Terrified, he immediately hastened to the
provost to obtain the release of the poor idiot.   He succeeded
after a great deal of trouble and at considerable expense—the
negotiations lasted till four o'clock.   But now, as he was

[1] Under the influence of the Black Death, he wrote his excellent tract :
" How One Should Learn to Die, and What Death is like without Preparation."

leaving the provost's house, he fell into the hands of the justice of the populace and was now forced to defend his own life. " The poisoner ! The murderer ! " the rabble howled. " His money has helped him with the provost, it won't help him with us ; kill him, throw him into the Rhine ! " " No," others exclaimed, " he would poison the river, he must be burnt." Then a huge peasant with a sooty jerkin and a long spear pushed his way through the crowd and said : " Listen, gentlemen, I will thrust my spear through the heretic, just as toads are speared ! Then we'll take off all his clothes, lift him up from behind with the spear and shove him into this thick hedge, so that he can't fall out. There the arch-villain can lie till the wind dries his bones and can be cursed by all who pass, so that he may be damned in this world and in the next ! " Suso heard and saw all this, but was unable to get in a word. The scene lasted so long that it began to grow dark. He walked up and down, besought each one individually to give him protection and shelter, but uncharitably he was repulsed from all doors, and the few good-hearted women who would have liked to have let him in did not dare. Thus the poor sufferer stood, deprived of all help, in the constant fear of death, waiting for the moment when they would seize him and kill him. Overcome by grief and weakness, he sank down by the hedge, raised his swollen eyes to heaven and prayed, submitting himself to the hands of God : " Those who would kill me are close by, my own heart is dumb with fear and unable to say whether it be more terrible to be burnt, drowned, or speared. O kind paternal heart, have mercy upon me." These last words of misery were reported to a priest in the neighbourhood, who hastened up with the necessary assistance and delivered him from the hands of the murderers, took him home for the night so that he might be safe for the moment, and next morning cleared up the whole matter.

Particularly in Germany all wells and springs were covered in at that time, so that no one should drink from them or prepare food with water taken from them. The inhabitants of innumerable towns and villages used exclusively rain and river water for a long time. In some places, for instance at Nuremberg, the leading citizens had wells sunk and bricked inside their houses. During one of the plagues in the Thirty

Years' War the inhabitants of Eschau (Main district), according to a popular legend, sank various wells, but everywhere the water showed a bluish colour and was plague water. When they wanted to sink a fifth well in the middle of the village there was a lack of hands to do the work, for the plague had already carried off so many. Just at that moment the first Swedes arrived in the place. As it was their intention to take quarters there for some time, perhaps also because the inhabitants were of their confession, they willingly offered their assistance. There water as pure and clear as any that had ever issued from the ground was found. They were, however, much afraid that the water might have been poisoned. But the Swedish captain said : " I will give you some good advice. Have the head of a Swede sculptured and attached to the well, then this water will never be poisoned. For the Swede is loved by God and feared by the Devil." The inhabitants did as he had told them—they had a stone column erected beside the well, and at the top of the column a head was carved to represent a Swede.

The rumour of the poisoned wells was by no means void of foundation. The water supply in the plains was drawn from open wells by means of buckets, or taken from the rivers at drawing stations established on bridges—a circumstance which explains that the inhabitants were constantly exposed to the danger of typhus, dysentery, and other epidemics. Now already at that time the Jews possessed so much medical knowledge as to avoid the use of well-water carefully in times of epidemics. This naturally aroused the greatest suspicions against them among the ignorant people. Tschudi, in his *Helvetian Chronicle*, reports the following :

" Many wise persons hold the opinion that the Jews are not guilty of poisoning the water, and that they only confessed it in excess of torture, but attribute the poisoning to the great earthquake which took place in January of last year, 1348; this burst open the crust of the earth and allowed the bad, noxious moistures and vapours to enter the wells and springs, as these impurities also fouled the air. This the Jews, of whom a large proportion are physicians and scientists, had learnt from their art and borne in mind, and on that account avoided the wells and springs, and in many places warned the

people against them.   For it would be impossible for them to
have poisoned all wells throughout Christendom.   In short,
the people were incensed against the Jews, and they could
expect no justice."

That the Jews should fall victims to the fantastic charge
of poisoning the wells was due less to religious or racial enmity
than to the accumulated hatred of capitalism among the
people.   Roscher rightly describes the great persecution of

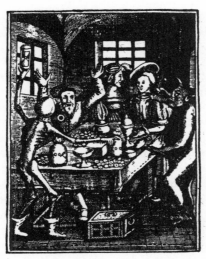

DEATH AND DEVIL FETCH A JEWISH
PROFITEER.
After Holbein.

the Jews in the fourteenth century as a financial crisis of a
barbaric nature, a mediæval form of what to-day we should
describe as a social revolution.   It is characteristic that
particularly the guilds, which must be regarded as social
institutions, hated and persecuted the Jews on account of
their privilege of enriching themselves by usury with great
ease.   Secular and particularly canonical laws prohibited the
Christian from taking interest, which was regarded as usury
from the earliest times of the Middle Ages.   As the Jews were
refused admission to the merchant guilds, they were excluded
from every participation in trade, and from the twelfth century

were practically restricted to financial enterprise, and as they were not bound by any canonical laws against usury, they became for every one—for princes, lords, municipalities, burghers, peasants—the real privileged money-lenders. The rate of interest about the middle of the fourteenth century varied between 21 and 86 per cent., and in individual cases rose from 127 to 166 per cent. In addition to this, in nearly all principalities and duchies the taxes and contributions had been farmed or pawned to Jews, who demanded what was due without regard for person. They had also suggested and imposed new taxes which were irksome to the subjects. The clergy were opposed to the Jews because they were increasing in the towns and reducing the incomes of the parishes. Besides, by letters of privilege granted by the princes, they were exempt from the far-reaching ecclesiastical jurisdiction. In the trading operations in which the clergy and monasteries engaged who were not always free of tax on their land, corn harvests and products, the Jews were less inclined to treat them with lenient consideration than the Christian tax-collectors, who were more or less dependent on them.

It was particularly by the clergy that the accusation was raised against the Jews that they murdered Christian children for the purpose of sacrifice, that they nailed them to a cross, and in derision of Christ played a mock passion. They were also said to have pounded consecrated hosts in mortars or to have pricked them with needles till they bled. Simon, the blessed child of Trent, of whom it was pretended that he had been murdered by the Jews at Easter in accordance with their rites, began after his burial to appear in miraculous revelations. From all Christian districts, pilgrimages were undertaken to the grave of the holy child, in whose honour a beautiful church was erected. At Zurich it was also maintained that a little boy had been found in 1349 who had been tortured to death by the Jews. He was entered, as a martyr and blood-witness of Christ, in the main cathedral, worshipped as a saint, and an altar erected above his grave. In the plague year 1401 the massacres of the Jews in Switzerland were again inaugurated by torturing a Jew till he confessed that he had purchased the blood of the child for three guilders. A sermon by the Dominican Johann Herold, who lived at Basle about 1425, shows to what extent the hatred and persecution of the Jews was carried by the clergy; in it he exhorts neither to eat nor to bathe with Jews, to let no houses to them, and to receive no presents from them. They are to fill no public office, to be forced to wear a distinctive dress, not to go in the streets in Holy Week and, on Good Friday, not to keep either doors or windows open. Christian workmen who work for them are to be excommunicated and will not be

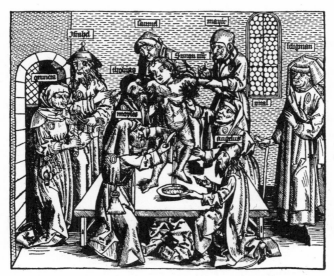

SIMON, THE BLESSED CHILD OF TRENT, BEING BUTCHERED
BY THE JEWS.
From Schedel's Chronicle.

buried in the churchyard, but in the knackers' field. Two girls were expelled from Zurich because they had intercourse with Jews. In other places girls were tied one on the top of the other and burnt (Swabian laws).

It is astounding to see the frankness with which the chroniclers, in spite of the general prevalence of anti-Semitism of the times, express themselves on the true reasons which led to the extermination of the Jews. Honest Fritsche actually calls the money of the Jews " the poison which brought their death," and Jacob Twinger adds : " If the Jews had been

poor, and rulers of the countries had not been in their debt,
they would never have been burnt." The chronicler of St.
Peter says, referring to the poisoning of the wells : " Whether
what they say be true or not, I do not know, but I believe
rather that the real cause was the great and incalculable
sums of money that the barons, together with the soldiers,
and the towns together with country people, had to pay them."
Klosener attributes the hatred of the nations for them to
their refusal to prolong credit. The same greed for money,
however, soon induced the towns and princes to recall the
Jews. The lack of the high taxes they had been paying had
so perceptible an effect that the kings, lords, and municipalities
vied with one another to reopen this closed source of income.
By the Golden Bull of 1355 Charles IV permitted the princes
" to keep Jews."

The heroism with which the Jews generally encountered
death did not fail to make an impression on the contemporaries.
When Markgrave Joachim of Brandenburg had had thirty-
eight Jews burnt on a grill, an eye-witness related some time
after : " These obstinate Jews (as would seem strange to me,
had I not seen it) heard the sentence with laughing mouths,
and greeted its execution with hymns of praise, and not only
did they sing and laugh on the grill, but for the most part
jumped and uttered cries of joy, and thus, in spite of the
evident wounds inflicted, suffered death with great firmness."
The clergy certainly explained this firmness as a work of the
Devil and the proof of extreme obstinacy. The devotion with
which the Jews nursed their co-religionists who fell sick of
the plague also made a great impression on many contemporaries. " It is unchristian," one author writes, and many
others express the same opinion, " that we refuse all help to
our neighbours. Turks and Jews do not behave thus, as, to
our shame, we must all confess. It is a great disgrace that
we who boast of being Christians and so well acquainted with
the Word of God should have to learn from non-Christians
and unbelieving Jews."

I will not treat of the persecutions of the Jews in plagues
of later dates. Again and again they were accused and put
to death in the most cruel manner. We will only cast a glance
at the insults hurled at the Jewish physicians who in times

of plague did extraordinarily good work. Owing to their knowledge of Arabic they possessed already in the fourteenth century an advantage over the northern physicians, who as yet had no translations from the Greek and Arabic. They played a particularly important rôle at Montpelier and Avignon, where they enjoyed special protection as physicians of the Pope. Although they had accompanied the Christians on their Crusades in 1338, at the Council of Aix Christians were forbidden to consult Jewish physicians. Pope Gregory made this prohibition so severe in 1581 that he not only imposed the most severe punishment on Jewish doctors who attended Christians, but refused the Sacrament and Christian burial to all Christians who should die under the care of Jewish physicians. Such attacks were certainly not of long duration. Municipalities and princes always had recourse to Jewish physicians, and they were even appointed as physicians-in-ordinary to some of the popes, e.g. Leo X, Clement VII, and Paul III. Particular difficulties were placed in the way of the Jewish physicians in Germany. In the sermons of the fifteenth and sixteenth centuries we are constantly encountering the prohibition to employ Jews as physicians. " That you should not think," says Geiler von Kaisersperg in one of his sermons, " that to accept the services of a Jew as a physician to regain your health is not a sin." " In the same manner there are some who run to the scurvy Jews and bring them their urine and ask their advice. But it is strictly forbidden to use any medicine prescribed by a Jew, except in cases where no other physician is available." As late as the year 1564 the appointment of a Jew as chief physician gave rise to a violent dispute at Thorn, the opponents asking " whether it was conscionable to appoint a blasphemer and vagrant to such a position."

The legend of Ahasver, the eternal wandering Jew, which originated in the thirteenth century, has always cropped up again in times of plague, until in 1602 it appeared in Germany in the form of a chap-book. It prompted Jean Paul to a very apt saying : " We have an eternal Jew, but where is the eternal Christian ? " Already in the fourteenth century there was a man who, free from all prejudice and inspired by true humanity, denounced the hatred of the Jews, as far as it was founded on a religious basis, as the excrescence of a restricted mind and intolerance in its most ugly form. This was Giovanni Boccaccio, who incorporated the story of the three rings in his *Decameron*, and by imparting a more delicate turn to it endowed it with the tendency of the equality of the three religions.

APPENDIX

A Letter from the Cologne Municipality—The Trial of Well-Poisoners at Chillon, 1348—Complaint of the Jews of Prague of their Boycott by Christian Physicians

Letter of the Municipality of Cologne which is directed to that of Strasbourg in the matter of the Jews, A.D. 1349. To the most cautious, etc., etc., at Strasbourg we, magistrates of Cologne, dispatch, etc.

Dear Friends,—In regard to the devastating epidemic of plague which unfortunately is spreading everywhere and raging already in many places, and in connexion with which all kinds of rumours are current concerning and accusing the Jews both in your town and in ours, so that it is openly asserted that this epidemic is attributable to the poisoning of the wells into which the Jews have thrown poison, we hear that serious complaints have been put forward against the Jews in some small towns and territories. In order to ascertain whether or not these rumours and complaints are well founded, we have addressed letters of enquiry to you and to other municipalities, but have received no satisfactory reply. Recently you reported to us that up to then you had been unable to penetrate to the bottom of the real state of facts. If now in the large towns prosecutions and executions of the Jews were to be instituted (which in our town we would not permit so long as we are able to prevent them, as long as we are convinced that the Jews are innocent of the atrocious deeds brought up against them), this procedure might give rise to great trouble and entail serious consequences. And if we are called upon to express our opinion in regard to this great plague, we must confess that we consider it to be a scourge of God, and consequently we shall permit of no prosecutions of Jews in our town on account of these rumours, but we shall protect them, as they were faithfully protected by our fore-fathers. We therefore urgently and amicably beseech you that, as in all matters you are accustomed to proceed with wisdom and caution, you will in this matter of the Jews be guided by justice and moderation, and for this purpose take measures in good time to prevent any risings of the people which might result in an indiscriminate slaughter of the Jews and involve other evils, and that to the best of your endeavours you will prevent the minds of the people being incited against the Jews, lest this excitement should spread to the towns of the Lower Rhine and penetrate to our district ; and you also may faithfully protect and defend the Jews in your town, as was done by your ancestors until such time when the full truth may be made known to you. For should, on account of the Jews, rioting break out with you, this would certainly not be without influence on other towns. It will, therefore, certainly be for the good if you and we and other large towns proceed with wisdom and caution in this matter. Should you by any chance have received new and reliable information from kings and princes, or from the Jews them-selves, let us receive them by this same messenger.

Dated this 12th day of January, A.D. 1349.

THE TRIAL OF WELL-POISONERS AT CHILLON, 1348

Reply of the Castellanus Chillionis to the Municipality of Strasbourg, together with a copy of the inquisition and confession of several Jews in *castro Chillionis detentorum, super facto tossici et veneni*, for poisoning, de Anno 1348.

To the Noble and Prudent Magistrates, Council and Community of the Town of Strasbourg, from the Castellian of Chillon, Deputy of the Lord Magistrate at Chablais. With submissive and respectful greetings. As I am given to under-stand that you are desirous of being made acquainted with the confession of the Jews and with the evidence brought against them, I therefore inform you and all of your friends who may be desirous of knowing by this present communication that the Bernese have received a copy of inquisitions and confessions of the Jews who were recently in their territory and were accused of having placed poison in the wells and in many other places, and that these accusations have proved quite true, as many Jews have been submitted to torture and some were exempted because they confessed and were brought before another court and burnt. Also Christians, to whom the Jews had given some of the poison, were placed on the wheel and tortured. The burning of the Jews and the reported torturing of the Christians took place in the county of Savoy.

Confessions of the Jews made in the year of the Lord, 1348, on September 15th, at the castle of Chillon, who had been arrested in the New Town concerning the poisoning of which they were accused, of wells and springs here and elsewhere, also of food and other things with the purpose of killing and extermining the whole of Christendom.

1. Balavignus the Jew, a surgeon and inhabitant of Thonon, although arrested at Chillon, as he was found within the Castle, was only placed on the rack for a short time, and when he had been taken off he confessed after some considerable time that about six weeks ago Master Jacob, who since Easter had been staying at Chambéry, in accordance with orders, and who had come from Toledo, sent him to Thonon by a Jew boy poison in an eggshell ; this was a powder in a thin sewn leather bag, together with a letter, in which he was ordered on pain of ban and in obedience to their law to put this same poison into the larger and smaller wells of his town, as much as was required to poison the people who fetched their water from there, and that he should reveal this to no one on pain of the above punishment. Further, in the same letter he was instructed to forward the same order to several other places by command of the Jewish Rabbis or masters of their law ; and he confessed that he had secretly placed the quantity of poison or powder indicated in a well on the lake shore near Thonon one evening beneath a stone. He confessed further that the above-mentioned boy had brought him more letters dealing with the same matter which were addressed to many other Jews, and particularly some were directed to

Mossoiet, Banditono and Samole to at Villeneuf,one to each, and others to Musseo Abramo and Aqueto of Montreux, to the Jews of Vevey, and others again to Benetono at St. Moritz and to his son ; further, others to Viviandus Jacobus, Aquetus and Musset, Jews at Moncheoli, and many other letters were borne by the boy, as he said, to various out-of-the-way places, but he could not say to whom they were addressed.   Further, he confessed that when he had placed the poison mentioned in the well at Thonon, he expressly forbade his wife and children to make further use of the well, but refused to tell them the reason.   He swore by his law and by all contained in the Pentateuch, in the presence of several reliable witnesses, that all he had confessed was entirely true.

Further, on the following day, Balavignus, in the presence of many reliable witnesses, of his own free will and without application of the rack, affirmed that the above-quoted confession was true, and repeated it word for word, and of his own free will confessed that one day coming from Thur, near Vevey, he placed a quantity of the poison wrapped in a rag of about the size of a walnut which had been given him by Aqueto of Montreux, an inhabitant of the above-mentioned Thur, in a well below Mustreuz, called the Fontaine de la Conerayde—that he had deposited this poison, he told and revealed to the Jew Mamssiono and his son Delosaz, inhabitants of Villeneuf, that they should not drink of the well ; he stated that the colour of the poison was red and black.

Further, on the 19th day of the month of September, the above-mentioned Balavignus confessed, without application of the rack, that the Jew Mussus of Villeneuf had told him three weeks before Whitsuntide that he had placed poison in his own well at Villeneuf, in the tollhouse, and that he no longer drank its water, but water from the lake.   He confessed, further, that this same Jew Mussus had told him that he had put poison in the tollhouse well at Chillon under the stones, of which well an examination was made and the above-mentioned poison found, of which a sample was given to a Jew, who died in consequence.   He further stated that the rabbis had ordered him and other Jews to refrain from drinking of the poisoned water for the first nine days after the placing of the poison.   Further, that as soon as he had placed the poison, as stated above, he immediately revealed it to the other Jews. He confessed, further, that, about two months ago, he had been at Evian and had discussed the matter with the Jew Jacob, and, among other things, asked him if he, like the others, had received a letter and poison. Jacob answered that he had. He asked him, further, if he had obeyed the order, and Jacob replied that he had not placed the poison, but had handed it to the Jew Saveto, who had placed it in the well de Morer at Evian, and he ordered him, Balavignus, that he should carry out carefully the instructions he had received. He said that Aqueto of Montreux had reported that he had placed some of the poison in the well above Thur, from which he had drunk several times at Thur. He confessed that Samolet had told him that he had placed the poison he had received in a well, but he refused to tell him which. Balavignus alleged, further, that as a surgeon he knew that if anyone was affected by this poison and anyone touched him in this condition, when overcome by weakness, he was sweating, that by this contact he might easily be infected, as also by the breath of anyone infected ; and of this he was convinced, as he had heard it from experienced medical men, and he was further convinced that the Jews could not deny these charges, as they were fully conscious that they were guilty of the actions with which they were charged. The said Balavignus was taken across the lake in a boat from Chillon to Clarens to verify and point out the well into which, as he alleged, he had placed the poison. When he arrived he was made to get out of the boat, and when he saw the place and the well where he had deposited the poison he said : " That is the well in which I put the poison." This well was examined in his presence, and the linen bag in which the poison was wrapped was found in the mouth of the well by a public notary, Heinrich Gerhard, in the presence of many people and was shown to the said Jew. He then admitted and confessed that this was the linen cloth in which the poison had been, and that he had placed it in the open well, and that it was parti-coloured, black and red. This linen cloth was taken away and is preserved as evidence. The said Balavignus admitted that all that he had narrated above was true to the last detail, and that he believed that this alleged poison contained some part of the basilisk, as he had heard say that the poison could not be prepared without basilisk, and of this he felt sure.

2. Banditono, a Jew of Villeneuf, was also on September 15th subjected to slight torture on the rack; afterwards, when taken off the rack, after a long time, he confessed that he had placed a quantity of poison, roughly of the size of a walnut, which had been given him by Mussus, a Jew, at Thur, near Vevey, in the well at Carutet to poison the gentiles.

Further, on the following day, the said Banditono, of his own free will and without torture, confessed and admitted that his previous statement was true, and further confessed that Master Jacob of Pasche, who hailed from Toledo and had settled at Chambéry, had sent him a supply of this poison, roughly of the size of a large nut, to Pilliex by a Jewish servant, together with a letter containing instructions that he was to put the poison in the wells on pain of ban. This poison he placed in the well Cecleti de Roch, it being contained in a leather bag. He confessed, further, that he had seen many other letters which the said servant was conveying, and which were addressed to Jews. He also saw that the said servant had delivered a letter to the Jew Samoleto at Villeneuf, above the upper gate outside the town. He further said that the Jew Massolet had informed him that he had placed poison in the well near the bridge at Vevey, to wit on the Evian side.

3. The said Mamsson, a Jew of Villeneuf, was on the above-mentioned 15th day of the stated month placed on the rack, he confessed nothing of the above-mentioned incidents, alleging that he knew nothing at all about them, but on the following day he admitted of his own free will and without the application of torture in the presence of many people that on a certain day in the Whit week of the previous year he and another Jew called Provençal of Moncheolo had been walking together and whilst walking the said Provençal had said to him : " It must be done. You must put the poison I am going to give you into that well, or woe betide you." And that was the well of Chabloz Cruez, between Vyona and Mura. He, Mamsson, took the quantity of poison, roughly the size of a nut, and placed it in the well, and he believed that

the Jews of the places round Evian had held a council among themselves concerning this poison business before Whitsuntide. Further, he alleged that the said Balavignus had one day revealed to him that he had placed poison in the well de la Conery, below Mustruez. Alleged further that none of the Jews could deny participation in this matter, as they were all implicated and guilty. The said Mamsson was on the following 3rd of October brought before the Commissioners and changed nothing in his statement, except that he had not himself placed poison in the well.

All this the above-mentioned Jews swore by their law before execution, stating that it was true, and all Jews above the age of seven were implicated, for they had all had knowledge of and were guilty of this matter.

[The other seven interrogations contained in the document differ from the above only in regard to the persons interrogated, and offering little variety. A characteristic place at the end of the document may therefore be quoted. The whole document speaks for itself.]

Dear Friends, when I received your communication and saw its purport I could not refrain from having the confessions of some Jews copied.

But there still remained many other accusations and proofs against the said Jews and others living in the county of Savoy which have been brought forward both by Jews and Christians, who have already suffered punishment for the exceedingly great crimes, which for the moment were not available and could not be forwarded. And you should be informed that all Jews resident at Villeneuf have been burnt by legal sentence. In August, three Christians were flayed for poisonings, at which execution I was present myself. At many other places also Christians have been arrested on the charge of such crimes. Particularly at Evian, Gebenne, Crusilien, and Hochstett, who finally with their last breath have admitted and confessed that they had received the poison they had laid from the Jews. Some of these Christians were quartered, some flayed, and some hanged. And commissions have been appointed by the authorities for the prosecution of the Jews, of whom I believe that none will be spared.

COMPLAINT OF THE JEWISH COMMUNITY AT PRAGUE IN THE
YEAR 1714, TOGETHER WITH THE REPLY OF THE MEDICAL
FACULTY

The community of the Jews have presented a complaint
to the Royal Court to the effect that medical men refuse to
attend patients in the Jewish quarter and to prescribe medicine for them. The Royal Government has communicated
this reply to the Lord Rector and the Academical Senate
with the comment : that as it was known that the danger
of infection has now entirely ceased, the public, on the other
hand, demands that vigilant watch should be kept that
nothing in any way liable to introduce such diseases should
be tolerated, the worshipful duly appointed Royal Government
does hereby order their Excellencies and Honours the Lord
Rector Magnificus and the Magistrates Academicus that they
should interrogate the medical faculty and from them demand
reasonable explanation why medical practitioners refuse to
visit the Jewish quarters and prescribe medicine for Jewish
patients, and forthwith report the nature of this explanation
to the Royal Governor.

Ex Consilo Regiae Cancellariae, Boh-Prague, die 14 *Junii,*
1714.

ADALBERT W. WANDAU.

Reply of the Medical Faculty.

Magnifice Domine Rector and worshipful Academical
Senate ! The supplication and complaint of the Jewish
Elders submitted to the most worshipful Royal Government
stating that the Doctors of Medicine have been forbidden to
visit in the Jewish quarter and there to treat patients, having
been remitted to us by you for report, we have on July 6th
summoned a medical council in which we had the complaint
of the Jews read and examined, and have ascertained that it
is an absolute untruth that the Doctors of Medicine have ever
been forbidden to attend the Jewish community and to
prescribe medicine for them, and it was ascertained that no
member of the faculty had any knowledge of any such prohibition, so that it cannot be deduced from the fact that some

doctors of medicine have refused to go to the Jewish quarters when called upon to do so. We, on the other hand, have full justification for complaint against the Jews that they practice deceit on the doctors, refuse correct information concerning their diseases, and secret other patients or dead persons, harbour foreign Jews, and have recourse to all kinds of quacks; only when these are of no further avail and hinder the patients in their recovery or render them incurable do they come to us to seek help, at a stage when we can no longer acquire the honour of healing. Besides it must not be left out of account that in the Jewish quarter, both in the public streets and the private houses, filth has become too prevalent and gives rise to such stench that one may easily feel repugnance to enter the Jewish quarter, so that it has frequently occurred that some of us who have gone there, on account of excessive stench, have returned with catarrh or other disease. And it is no wonder if from such filth and stench the people are attacked by various diseases or infected by an epidemic of the plague. Further, the pharmacies in the Jewish quarter are badly stocked, and the apothecaries so inexperienced that they are incapable of compounding a prescription, and consequently their medicines can have no proper effect.

This reply we beg to submit to the worshipful Academical Senate with the submissive request that they may be pleased to suggest to the most worshipful Royal Government the advisability of instituting an enquiry concerning the vagabonds and immoral elements harboured by the Jews. With which we beg to take leave and remain,

The worshipful Academical Senate's most obedient,
MEDICAL FACULTY OF THE CARLO-FERDINAND
UNIVERSITY OF PRAGUE.

This document was forwarded by the worshipful Academical Senate to the Royal Government.

TERRIBLE TESTAMENT OF A CHRISTIAN PROFITEER

A profiteer stricken by the plague has left a most terrible last will and testament. The man was originally an artisan, but under pressure of his proud wife he abandoned his handicraft and took to trade. " In this, although with a bad conscience and by means of all kinds of tricks and financial dodges, he had grown rich, so that together with his wife he led a luxuriant life and was able to outshine all his friends and neighbours. When finally God threw him on a bed of sickness, and as he grew worse and worse, his wife, children, and friends in the presence of his confessor exhorted him to make his last will and testament. At last he consented, sent for notaries and witnesses, and dictated the following terrifying words : ' My body I leave to the earth, my soul I bequeath to the devil ; furthermore the souls of my wife, my children, and my confessor. My own soul, because without regard to right or justice I have on every possible occasion ruthlessly scraped together all I could ; that of my wife, because for the satisfaction of her pride she has incited me to do so ; those of my children because to enrich them I have impoverished others ; that of my confessor, because, while sharing the luxuries of my table, he has never reminded me of my sins, nor rebuked me for them.' "

Another author gives a more detailed account of the will, which he says was taken down as follows : " First I leave my body to the earth, but my soul to the devil in hell." His wife was terrified and said : " But, dear husband, what are you doing ? Think of God, the Almighty ! " But he said : " I know what I am about. To whom should I leave my soul when dying but to him whom I have served all my life ? I have never had any dealings with God ; I have no reason to believe that he would care to have me." He then continued to dictate : " And you, my wife, must accompany me to the devil, for by your proud disposition you have been the cause why for the sake of money and possessions I have given myself to the devil. If you agreed to the one, you must consent to the other." He said nothing about the children. But in regard to the confessor he continued as follows. And when the confessor expostulated with him he said : " And you, miserable parson, must come along with us, for you have been at my table every day and have seen the unchristian manner of my life, but have never rebuked me for it, but considered high living and profiteering as of greater importance than my poor soul, which, in the time of my life, you might have rescued from the claws of the devil. As you are so enamoured of my society, you shall in all eternity remain at my table ; and as you enjoyed my temporal well-being on earth, you shall share with me the eternal torment of hell." Thereupon he died with many a sigh, having before expiring cried several times : " What availeth me now all my great magnificence ? What availeth me now my riches and all my pride ? "

CHAPTER IX

THE EROTIC ELEMENT IN THE PLAGUE

Licentiousness in all classes—Erotic frescos in the cathedrals—The Fraternity of the Free Mind—The Accademia d'amore—Fever delirium—Plague societies—Ecclesiastic war on sexuality—Marriage mania—The wife returned from the grave—Syphilis and plague—Plague spreading by amorous women—Don Juan and Tannhaeuser—Giorgione's death—Petrarch's Laura.

Appendix : Description of the plague in Florence in the year 1527 by Nicolo Machiavelli.

BEFORE the outbreak of the Black Death the general dissolution of morality had already reached a very high degree. " From the greatest to the most insignificant," Boccaccio reports, " bishops, prelates, and temporal lords worshipped voluptuousness in the most disgraceful manner, and abandoned themselves not only to natural but also to unnatural lust without shame or restraint, so that by the influence of harlots, male and female, the most important things could be obtained from them." But in middle-class society, up till then, a certain appearance of respectability had been preserved ; this too had disappeared after the terror of the Black Death had swept away not only all law courts and police, but had destroyed the last conventions of decency. " Without heed of what is decent or indecent the people live only guided by their own instincts, and do by day or night, alone or in company, whatever their inclination may prompt them. And it is not only the laity who behave thus, but the nuns in the convents also, neglecting their rules, abandon themselves to carnal lust, and deem that by voluptuousness and excess they will prolong their lives."

As once in Athens, many in Florence were now convinced that for reasons of health it was incumbent to lead as dissolute a life as possible " The most reliable medicine, they maintained, was to drink extensively and to have a good time, to wander about with song and merriment, satisfying, as far as possible, every desire, and to laugh and jeer at what was bound to come." In Corsica, in 1355, one party introduced the community of women and goods, and represented this to the Corsicans as the advent of the golden age. In Rome, during the plague, brilliant festivals and drunken revels were held. Everyone kept open-house not only for his friends, but particularly for strangers. In the same way in Paris, balls, banquets, sports, and tournaments formed a continuous sequence. " The French, so to say, danced on the corpses of their relations. It was actually as if they wished to display their joy at the upset in their houses and at the death of their friends." The bas-reliefs and capitals in the French churches are of extraordinary interest ; they represent erotic scenes. In the cathedral of Alby a fresco even depicts sodomites engaged in sexual intercourse. That homo-sexuality was also well known in parts of Germany is proved by the trials of the Beghards and Beguins in the fourteenth century, particularly by the confessions of the brethren Johannes and Albert of Bruenn which are preserved in a Greifswald manuscript. From these it is evident that the Brethren of the Free Mind did not consider homo-sexuality as sinful. " And if one brother desires to commit sodomy with a male, he should do so without let or hindrance and without any feeling of sin, as otherwise he would not be a Brother of the Free Mind." In a Munich manuscript we read : " And when they go to confession and come together and he preaches to them, he takes the one who is the most beautiful among them all and does to her according to his will, and they extinguish the light and fall one upon the other, a man upon a man, and a woman upon a woman, as it just comes about. Everyone must see with his own eyes how his wife or daughter is abused by others, for they assert that no one can commit sin below his girdle. That is their belief." The other curious doctrines that incest is permissible, even when practised on the altar, that no one has the right to refuse consent, that Christ risen from the dead had intercourse with Magdalena, etc., all indicate that such deterioration and confusion of moral ideas was only caused by the great plagues, particularly by that of 1348. In England, where immorality had also attained a high degree, the ladies appeared at the great tournaments in male attire with a sword at their sides. During the plague at Milan in 1586 the " Political Chamber Fraternities" were formed; they spent the whole day "with all kinds of games at cards, dice and the like, and also with bestial amusements and over eating and drinking." The "Accademia d'amore" became celebrated: it was a company of young nobles who in imitation of Decamerone retired to a castle and there spent the days with stories, games, and the pleasures of love. The chroniclers of those days report with evident satisfaction that the plague mocked at the moats and drawbridges of that castle and made a thorough clearance among those " worldly excrescences and sinful worldly felines."

Several circumstances and accompanying features of the plague tended to stimulate sexual desire. In the rhymed chronicle of Geoffroy de Paris we already read of the plague year 1315 :

> La nuit, gisoient toutes nues
> Les bonnes Genz par les rues.

And in later times of plague it is reported that at night, or even in daytime, women ran about the streets in shameless nakedness. Although these were certainly cases of fever' delirium, this involuntary prostitution was certainly inducive of much immorality. Another seducive element was the circumstance that the healthy people of both sexes in many cases formed small plague societies and lived promiscuously, often in restricted space, during the duration of the plague. In Germany just at that time it became customary to go to bed entirely without night clothing. Finally the great riches inherited suddenly and unexpectedly by many seduced to extravagances of all kinds. The poor, too, had become accustomed to indolence and led a life of carelessness. In consequence of the lack of man power, workmen were so much in demand that, for instance, in Brandenburg after the plague years 1502–1504, the workmen earned so much in two days that they could live on it for the rest of the week.

That there is no power on earth so irresistible as that of Eros is fully borne out by the experience of plague times. Kundmann relates the following :

" In the large, beautiful village of Netsch the plague was
raging most violently, on account of which, in order that the
disease should not spread to the still uninfected villages, these
placed vigilant guards day and night for their protection.
Now it happened that a young agricultural labourer from
Stampen was among the guards and was violently enamoured
of a peasant wench at Netsch. As this girl was attacked by
the plague and her sweetheart heard of it, he resolved to bid
her good-night before she passed into the other world. On
this account he left his post during the night, ran into the
infected village and approached his sweetheart so close that
he returned with a boil in the same place in which she had had
one. Now, he had carried this out so secretly that if what he
had left in the wench's belly had not betrayed the matter, it
would have remained unknown. In the meanwhile the lad fell
sick in his watchman's hut, went home to his father's house,
infected it with the plague and returned to his hut. As soon
as it was observed that there was illness in his father's house
and the son was sick in his hut, a guard was set both on the
house and on the son in his hut, but the whole house died out,
and only he who had caused the whole evil escaped."

" At Ludwigsdorf, which is situated not far from Oels, the
plague was also raging most violently ; a young peasant
wench was attacked. So soon as her sweetheart heard of it,
he went to see her in the night and indulged so long in amorous
sport till he brought home a plague boil as a reward. But
this had not been done so secretly that the parents of both the
girl and the lad had not noticed it, and although both pairs of
parents rebuked their children with harsh words for this
crime, they could not prevent this pair of lovers from coming
together every night, now in one place, now in another, and
mutually squeezing out their plague boils. Dr. Eggerdes
happened to come to the place where the parents of these two
lovers were, and they begged him for God's sake to permit
them to fetch a priest from Oels to marry their children before
they died in their sins, as they were both infected by the
plague and yet could not be restrained from coming together
every night and doing that which they had no right to do.
And a few days before their boils had actually burst. The
doctor replied to the mother : ' As your children's boils have

burst and they are still so strong that they can go to meet each other and indulge in amorous sport, they will certainly not die of the disease.' "

Abraham a Santa-Clara, in his pamphlet *Merk's Wein*, is a classical example of how the ecclesiastics in whom the true mediæval spirit survived, availed themselves of the plague to combat sexuality which they hated violently :

" Come here, ye worldly apes, face-loving fools. Venus champions, come with me to several places in Vienna, where huge trenches have been filled with corpses; just contemplate what you have adored, to what you have paid so many compliments, given more flattery than was lavished on Egyptian cats, with what you drove to the pleasure gardens, there in the cool grottos by the clear water sullied your own consciences, what frequently you clothed in red robes and dresses and in return deprived of the white of innocence ; look at what robbed you of sheep and sleep, of peace and plenty, of science and conscience: come here, and gaze into the graves in which so many thousands lie. There she lies who charmed you with her crinkly curls—now they are but lousy mats and no longer powdered with musk, but stuck together with matter and dirt like a dried-up varnish-brush ; behold there she who with her magnetic eyes attracted your heart, the clearness of whose eyes you valued more than diamonds—now they lie sunken in her head and are but hollows made for worms to nest in ; look, take away that handkerchief from your nose, so that you may the better see there the roses of her whose cheeks often converted you into a golden butterfly. Follow me still farther; there is another trench and in it lie many thousand persons like pickled game in a barrel, solely with the difference that instead of salt quicklime is used. Behold there her whose ruddy lips were sweeter to you than sugar-candy—now the quicklime has consumed these delicacies, that now the teeth grin out like those of a snarling dog on its chain. Come here and gaze on that which has enticed you, charmed you, maddened you, delighted you ; what was your pleasure, all that is now a stinking mass, a confused heap, a conglomeration of filth, a bait for worms, a repulsive heap of matter. Take but one handkerchief full of this stench home with you and meditate what it means for such an abomination to suffer for all eternity. Oh, for all eternity!—think how many such a green wench must feel who used to lie in your arms and is now in the burning pitch of hell ! Oh, what repentance would overcome such a miserable dupe, if once more she could escape ; but no, it is in vain—for all eternity, eternity, eternity ! O Eternity, eternally forever, eternally never, never to escape for all eternity ! ever to remain there for all eternity ! "

Nearly all physicians and plague authors warn earnestly against matrimonial relations, in the first place on account of the extraordinary danger of infection and then because they consume the strength and render the body liable and prone to attract the disease. *In peste Venus pestem provocat*, i.e. " In times of plague the sport of Venus invites the plague," was proverbial. " And there is nothing that predisposes the body more to the plague than lasciviousness. This too the reason why the newly married, because more prone to sexual excesses, are easily infected. It was due to this that, during the plague at Nimeguen, for many bridegrooms on the second or third day after marriage mortuary candles had to be burnt instead of the nuptial torch, and on this account it is altogether wrong to give wives to young men, but still worse to give them to old men." In spite of these wise warnings, marrying mania raged and the plague acted like a clever matchmaker. An acquaintanceship of twenty-four hours was considered sufficient foundation for the conclusion of a matrimonial bond. Widows whose faces were still stained with the tears at the loss of their recently dead husbands were seen to take comfort with a new husband who in the course of a few days was again torn from their sides. Particularly among the lower classes the marrying mania assumed fantastic proportions. Enriched by undreamt-of wages or unexpected inheritance, quite old maids formed nuptial alliances, and quite young men put marriage rings on the fingers of toothless hags. Even sick people whose plague boils were still running satisfied their desire for matrimonial joys by marriage. " A woman at Nimeguen in six weeks married three men. The priest must have recognised her and lent a helping hand. But Diemerbrock recommends the following treatment : that a harlot scourger should cleanse the lascivious cow of her maternity mania (*furor uterinus*) with keen rods." Cornarius is not of this opinion ; he says

" that as so many men had fled from the plague, the women could find no satisfaction and were thus left to vain desire, which was the real reason why so many women died of the plague." He also quotes an example of how the plague was healed by venereal lasciviousness : " Such things occurred in the year 1636 during the plague in Holland, where a servant lying sick of the plague, having in three places of her body carbuncles and fiery boils, had intercourse with a young man, her lover, who came to her every night in the garden in which she had been lodged and without inflicting harm upon the young man recovered. Which story was narrated by a good poet in a fine ballad which on account of its pleasing and clever character was printed at Hamburg."

Rondinelli, in his history of the plague at Florence, relates an amusing case : A woman who had been buried with several plague corpses recovered from her coma, got out of the grave and returned home to her husband, who was expecting anything but this. He treated her as a ghost and drove her away, shouting after her that his wife was well and thoroughly dead. Full of horror at her reception, the unfortunate woman went to Rondinelli's grandfather, who knew her well and who pleaded for her with her husband until he received her. " One is not so incredulous," Rondinelli adds, " if one really loves."

Peter Bayle relates a case of connubial love. When Theodor Koornhert was cast into prison for heresy, his wife, imagining that he would not be set free again, is said to have endeavoured to catch the plague and to infect him with it, so that they might die together. Koornhert, however, was liberated, and fortunately his wife's endeavours were not successful. Most remarkable things are related by many plague authors of the excesses of lepers. Thus at Nuremberg the feeding of the sick (by which the lepers are meant) was discontinued, because they had become quite lascivious, and one of them molested a beautiful woman in the public street with his affection. " The hot blood of this lascivious goat," it is stated, " was cooled by the headman's sword." The same is reported of syphilists. Several physicians claim to have observed that no one suffering from venereal disease was ever attacked by the plague. Friedrich Schreiber says in his experiences and thoughts of the plague : " Is not the plague a most rapid form of venereal disease ? And is not venereal disease a slow plague ? It makes no difference that the two veritable plagues in regard to rapidity are so different from one another, the seat of both diseases is the same, the pale membranes, the water vessels and water glands ; in the consequences of both are the same curdling of the water in the blood producing either cold gangrene or slow-creeping hot gangrene."

A Tartar physician reports on a remarkable manner of producing the plague which was practised by women belonging to the lower nobility at Bucarest in the eighteenth century. They understood the art " when in the country for a short time of amusing themselves without their husbands, particularly when urgent financial consideration rendered it necessary. For, as they did not possess the means to get themselves up like the most aristocratic ladies and yet wished to vie with these, their lovers were frequently obliged to make considerable contributions. And as in town it was not so easy to deceive their husbands, close friends arranged at social gatherings when and where they would make a plague. For this purpose a gipsy woman or some other poor person was necessary of whom it was maintained that she had died of the plague—a report which these women by means of their connexions spread far abroad in a very short time. Everyone who can retires to the villages at the general alarm, with the exception of the noblemen who are retained in town by their service. And now the good wives can live with their lovers as long as they deem expedient."

Thomas Plater, in his autobiography, gives an impressive example of mediæval charity which survived, perhaps, longer than elsewhere in Germany, where especially the Black Death had stimulated the deep meditations of the mystics on things that were of eternal value for humanity. When Plater was seeking a shelter for his master, who while travelling had fallen ill of the plague, he was refused roughly everywhere. "After some refreshment I simply went from one house to the next and begged only for a shed in which he could die, for I could see that he would not live long. At last I found a woman who was about to be delivered ; the midwives had been to see her three times. The woman wept, she felt such compassion for the man for whom I was begging the people so fervently and at the same time offering sufficient compensation. She said, ' Go, my good fellow, bring your master to me.' The woman hailed from Basle. I then went and hired a woman to help me bring him from the inn, about the distance of a stone's throw, but I had to pay her half a guilder. As we were leading him to the house, the peasants stood on both sides and peered at us. I gave them a good talking to and reproached them for their coldness of heart. When I brought him to the house, the woman had prepared an arm-chair and we placed him in it before the door that he should rest a little. She gave him some broth and he ate two spoonfuls; then the woman kissed him on the mouth and wept for pity, for he was a fine big man and well dressed. Then we took him to a little bedroom where a nice bed had been prepared. There she again gave him some broth and again kissed him, weeping."

Among the educated in Latin countries during the fourteenth century which produced the two most celebrated European legends, that of Don Juan and that of the knight Tannhaeuser, sensuality had become entirely emancipated from religion, whereas the increasing belief in devils and witches among the uneducated classes proved how keen and unavailing the contest against sexuality, which had been repressed so long, had become. In the *Decamerone*, which was written between 1348 and 1358, we are confronted with the erotic conception of the Quattrocento with all its joy in the downright sensual and unconcealed. The comforts of the Church have no place in this book, whereas that part of the human anatomy by which a certain Pope was in the habit of swearing, and of which, when he was reproached, he is said to have replied: "*È pero il padre di tutti i Santi*" (And yet it is the father of all the saints), is greeted with exultation and praised in song in a quite heathen manner.

A very strong description of the erotic emotion during the plague is supplied by Machiavelli in his narrative of the plague at Florence in 1527. Church and religion are subjected to derision, and his narrative concludes by his being seized during the requiem service by a deep passion for a beautiful woman.

An example of how love laughs at the fear of death is further the story which Vasari relates of Giorgione's death. At one of his garden parties at which he used to entertain his friends with music he is said to have become acquainted with a woman for whom he was seized with a deep love. " And both were exceedingly happy in their love." When his lady-love was attacked by the plague, Giorgione continued visiting her as usual, and together with her kisses received her mortal disease, of which he died in a short time.

All beautiful and noble women carried off by the plague have been incorporated in Petrarch's " Laura," one of the imperishable characters of the literature of the world, in which the great marvellous qualities of the female sex have been collected by the poet's power of combination.

APPENDIX

DESCRIPTION OF THE PLAGUE AT FLORENCE IN 1527
By Nicolo Machiavelli.

I hardly dare to apply my trembling hand to the page to begin so woeful a story ; the more I reflect on the great misery in my mind, the more repugnance do I feel to its terrible description. My eyes have seen it all and yet the narrative once more draws tears of pain from me. I know not where to begin and fain would once more lay down my pen. But the ardent desire to know if you are still alive causes me to over-come all trepidation. Our pitiful Florence now looks like nothing but a town which has been stormed by the infidels and then forsaken. One part of the inhabitants, who, like you, have fled from the deadly plague, have retired to the distant country houses; one part is dead, and yet another part is dying. Thus the present is torment, the future menace, so we contend with death and only live in fear and trembling. The clean, fine streets which formerly teemed with rich and noble citizens are now stinking and dirty ; crowds of beggars drag themselves through them with anxious groans and only with difficulty and dread can one pass through them. Shops and inns are closed, at the factories work has ceased, the law

courts are empty, the laws are trampled on. Now one hears
of some theft, now of some murder. The squares, the market
places on which the citizens used frequently to assemble, have
now been converted into graves and into the resort of a wicked
rabble. Men walk alone, and instead of meeting a friend one
meets plague sufferers. If by chance relations meet, a brother
a sister, a husband a wife, they carefully avoid each other.
What further words are needed ? Fathers and mothers avoid
their own children and forsake them. The one holds flowers,
another odoriferous herbs, a third a sponge, a fourth a glass, a
fifth small balls composed of various drugs in his hand, or
rather he holds them continuously to his nose ; they are his
means of protection. A few provision stores are still open,
where bread is distributed, but where in the crush plague boils
are also spread. Instead of conversation, which in the squares
was honourable, and profitable in the markets, one hears now
only pitiful, mournful tidings—such a one is dead, such a one is
sick, such a one has fled, such a one is interned in his house,
such a one is in hospital, such a one has nurses, another is
without aid, such-like news which by imagination alone would
suffice to make Æsculapus sick. Many seek the causes of the
evil. Some say : the astrologers threatened us with it.
Others, the prophets have predicted it. Signs and wonders
are recalled. The weather is blamed and the air which is said
to teem with plague infection, and that it was also so in 1348
and 1478. And thus many other things are said, so all unanimously agree that not only this evil but innumerable others
will bring down destruction on us. Although with a single
word I could put our deplorable home before your mind's eye,
by saying imagine it quite different and in every respect the
contrary of what you used to see it, and nothing could supply
you with a better report than this comparison, yet you shall
be able to gain a better insight into it, as imagination can
never supply so clear an impression as reality. But I cannot
depict the reality better than by taking my own life as a
specimen, and will, therefore, describe to you the manner in
which I live, so that in accordance with that you may image
the life of all the rest.

Know then on weekdays, at the hour when the sun dis-
perses the exhalations which rise from the earth, I leave my

house and proceed to my usual business, having before taken some medicine and a certain antidote against the poisonous disease, in which I place no slight confidence, although our excellent Mingo calls it a paper armour. Hardly am I a hundred paces from my house when every other thought, however serious and important, is expelled from my mind, for the first objects which as propitious presage strike my eye are the gravediggers, not those for the plague stricken, but the usual ones. As formerly they used to complain of too few deaths, they now complain of too many. Such great abundance would appear to cause want with them. Who would ever have thought that a time would come when they would wish for the recovery of a sick man, as they swear that they now seriously do. I am quite willing to believe it, for if those sick of the plague were to die at any other time or of some other disease, they would reap their usual profit.

When I then pass by the Monastery of San Miniato up to the towers where formerly I was nearly deafened by the noise of the beetles of the wool beaters and their rough conversation, I am now received by an uncanny silence. I pursue my way and in the neighbourhood of the New Market I encounter the plague on horseback which the first time I saw it really deceived me. For as from afar I saw borne by four white horses (so exactly of snow whiteness) a litter, I thought it must be a beautiful lady or a member of some great house. But when, instead of being accompanied by cavaliers, I saw it attended by the servants of St. Maria Nova, there was no need to make further enquiries.

But for me this was not sufficient and, so as to be able to give you a detailed account of everything on the morning of the first of the merry month of May, I entered the magnificent venerable church of St. Reparta. There were only three priests there—the one was singing a Mass, the second was acting as choir and organ, the third to hear confessions sat down on a seat surrounded by a wall in the middle of the first nave. In spite of this he had fetters on his feet and handcuffs on his wrists. This had been prescribed by the Vicarius so that in such great solitude he might resist the canonical temptations. Of pious women who were attending the Mass there were three—old women in hooded cloaks, hunchbacked, perhaps

lame, and each one was kneeling isolated in a separate pew
I believed that I recognised one as my grandfather's nurse.
Of pious men there were also three, who, without ever catching
sight of one another, hobbled on crutches round the choir,
casting the while looks of longing love at the three beauties.
Incredible, forsooth, had I not seen it with my own eyes.

Thus I remained quite astonished as one who does not
trust his own eyes, and as I believed that the people, as usual,
on the morning of this high feast day would teem to the tournament in the square, in this hope I partook myself there and
saw, instead of a tournament of men and horses, one of crosses,
biers, coffins, and tables, on which I saw corpses borne by the
gravediggers, who had been summoned by the Barlaccio, for
want of better, as sponsors for the high and mighty signors
who were just making their solemn entrance. I am inclined
to believe that if the number of the living did not suffice the
names of the dead were made to serve and called out according
to custom, although none of them had the luck of Lazarus.

As this spectacle did not strike me as either very imposing
or safe, I did not tarry long, and as I had no reason to believe
that in any other part of the town a larger company of noblemen were to be found, directed my steps towards the celebrated
square of St. Croce. Here I saw an immense dance of gravediggers, who were singing: " Welcome, plague; welcome,
plague." This was their merry " Welcome, May "; the sight
of them and the disharmony of their song and its words were
as painful to both my eyes as formerly the chant of the honourable maidens had been pleasing ; so that without hesitation I
took refuge in the church.

Here I said my usual prayer without noticing a single
witness, when from afar I heard a dismal, lamentable sound.
Approaching it I saw stretched out on the fresh graves, clad
in mourning weeds, a pale, grieved maiden, whose appearance
was more that of a corpse than of a living being. She was
bedewing her cheeks with bitter tears, and now tearing the
black tresses of her beautiful dishevelled hair, now beating her
bosom and her face with her own hands, so that it would have
moved a stone. Grief and pain came over me beyond all
measure, but I approached cautiously with the words : " Why
do you mourn so much ? " She quickly hid her face with the

hem of her dress, so that I should not recognise her. This naturally increased my curiosity. But the fear that she might be infected by the plague impeded my steps, but yet I told her she should not be afraid of me, I wished to give her advice and help. When bent down by her grief she wept, I added that I would not go away until I had seen her. Although for a short time she still hesitated, like a sensible and courageous lady she resolved to disclose herself to me. " How foolish I am," she said; " I did not flinch in the face of a whole people and should now be afraid of a single man who in my need wishes to assist me ? " By her dress and the excess of her passion she was disfigured, so that I recognised her more by her voice than by her form. I asked her the cause of her great grief. " Woe to me, unhappy woman," was her reply, " I cannot conceal it. I mourn the loss of all my happiness, and, should I live to the age of a hundred years, I can never again be happy. My greatest grief is that I, too, cannot die. I do not complain of the plague but of my own sad fate—that the unbreakable tie of love that with such art and care I had bound to a knot should be torn asunder, that I might not die with him, that here on the grave of my unlucky much beloved my tears should flow. Oh, with what pleasure did I so often enfold him in these once so happy, but now so miserable, arms ! With what delight did I gaze into his beautiful, shining eyes. With what longing did my greedy lips suck his fragrant mouth ! With what tenderness did I press my burning bosom against his warm, white, youthful breast. Oh, with what bliss did we so frequently meet to enjoy the supreme happiness of those who love, did we swim encircled by inextinguishable ardour in a sea of ecstasy."

Hardly had she pronounced these words when she sank unconscious to the ground, so that my hair stood on end lest she should be dead. Her eyes were closed, her lips discoloured, her face still paler than it was before. But the motion of her grief-laden bosom seemed to betray some slight trace of life. I began, as bound by common charity, to rub her body carefully, unlacing her in front, although she was not tightly laced, and laying her now one side, now on the other. So I applied all means which are generally used to restore vanished animation. At last I succeeded so far that she opened her weary eyes, and heaved so hot a sigh that, had I been of wax, I should have melted. I now endeavoured to encourage her. " O foolish, unhappy girl," I said, " why do you remain here still ? If your parents, your neighbours, or your acquaintances had found you here, what would they have said ? Where is your prudence, where your respectability ? " " Alas ! poor me," she replied, " the former I never possessed and the latter I lost with the dear glance of the beautiful eyes which was as necessary to me as water for the fish." " If, Donna, my advice has any value in your estimation," I replied, " I must entreat you to come with me—not for love of me, for of this I am unworthy, but for the sake of your own honour, which will soon be clean again, although at present it may be slightly tarnished, more by malicious tongues than by your fault. How many ladies do I know who have run away from their husbands and found refuge with others than their parents ! How many have been surprised by their relations and neighbours when they had very much forgotten themselves who to-day are deemed good and virtuous ? Truly to err is human, only one must be capable of finding the way back to one's virtuous self. If in future your conduct is satisfactory, you will find, rely on it, that it will soon be said that you had been basely slandered." In this manner I persuaded her, and led her back with me to her house.

The sun had already attained the centre of the sky and the shadows were growing shorter, when solitary, as always, I sat down to my meal. After a short rest I started off again to wander through the town, and directed my steps towards the new church of the Holy Ghost, where no signs for the preparation of divine service were evident, although it was the hour. The few friars who were present were walking angrily up and down the church, and assured me that a great many of them were already dead and that still more would follow, for they were not allowed to go out and had no store of provisions. I need hardly say that they set the church ablaze with curses; I think it must have been that their dead should not have to find their way out in the dark. I therefore quickly went away again—urged more by the fear of heaven than by dread of the disease, the friars repeated their blessings so frequently.

As I was now returning through the May street, as it was the calends of May, I did not find a single trace that might have reminded me of May. On the other hand, on the bridge I found a dead man, whom no one dared to approach, and when I entered the old church of the Holy Trinity I only found one single man. He seemed to be of nobility. I asked him what retained him in town, exposed to such great danger, and received the answer: "The love of my native town which has been forsaken by all its less-loving sons." I replied that he was doing much less wrong who sought to preserve himself for his native town, so as later on to be able to serve it than he who without benefiting it exposed himself to the danger of having to leave it for ever. "If then I may tell the truth to a sensible man," he replied, "so know it is not my native town, but that inconsolable lady whom you see kneeling there so piously who retains me—for her I am prepared to sacrifice my life."

It seemed to me that his mature age would have agreed better with a little less ardour, and I therefore remarked that at such times fathers forsook their children, wives their husbands. "My love," he replied, "is so great that it exceeds any degree of blood relationship, and if to avoid the plague cheerfulness is the best means, there is in the presence of my lady love a great joy, and away from her I should feel such grief that it alone would suffice to cause me bitter death. As you have found me solitary here, my love is also of a unique nature, and if you are in love and wish to live, remain near her whom you love. If you are not, follow my example and fall in love if you wish to escape the plague. You have still time." As I consider love in so far an even more devastating plague, as it is of longer duration, this conversation did not edify me and without saying more I went.

On the now-forsaken terrace of Spini I once more encountered the venerable father Fra Messio, who, perhaps to flee the plague, had left his monastery and was perhaps waiting here to confess one of his penitents outside the church. From him I learnt that in the venerable church of S. Maria Novella, of such beautiful construction, from which, on account of his good behaviour, he had been excluded, owing to the loving instruction of the worthy charitable brethren, more ladies were assembled than in any other church. I took him with me, although not much in accordance with his own desire, for the good friar seemed to fear what would certainly have happened to him if he had gone there without me. Nor did he remain long, and he had hardly made a slight bow before the altar, for he never suffered from excess of piety, when he went out, and, I think, returned to his business on the terrace.

I remained to hear the pleasing Compline of the brethren. Although I did not, as usual, see the large number of beautiful ladies and of grand gentlemen who assemble to admire their angelic faces and their divine manner of wearing their rich tasteful dresses, which, in conjunction with the sweet music, inspire much more to the game of love than to thoughts of heaven; yet I found there less solitude than in any other place, and believed I had discovered the reason why this church is rightly considered more favoured and blessed than any other. I, therefore, determined to remain till the end. In addition to me, although it was already evening, perhaps like me to hear the Completorium, a beautiful young lady in widow's weeds had remained there, to describe whose beauty would be an undertaking exceeding my powers. In order to give you some idea I will not remain quite silent about it, and what is lacking in my narration you may supply with your imagination.

In the first place and that could be seen at the first glance, although she was seated on the marble steps in the vicinity of the large chapel, reposing as if fatigued and supporting her somewhat pale face with her white arm, she was of the stature proper for a woman of fine figure. From this could be concluded that all parts of her body were in such fine proportion that, divested of her mourning clothes, they would have appeared to my eyes in marvellous beauty. This part, however, I will leave to your powers of imagination to reproduce, and will only describe what I had the happiness to discover. Her fresh charming flesh seemed ivory, and so soft and tender that the slightest touch would leave a trace behind no less than on the tender little dewy blade of grass on the green meadow the track of the small insect remains visible. Her eyes were like two burning stars, and from time to time she lifted them with such grace that one believed that in them one could see the heavens open. Her serene brow of the most just proportions was so clear and shining that insipid Narcissus, reflecting his own image in it as well as in the limpid spring, might have become enamoured of himself. Below it the finely traced arches of the black eyebrows formed a covering for the beautifully gleaming eyes, around which Amor was constantly hovering playfully and from whence he dispatched his arrows, wounding now this and now some other loving heart. Her ears, to judge from that part of them which was visible, were small, round, and of such form that every physiognomist must have declared them a sign of great intelligence. What shall I say of the tender honey mouth between two cheeks on which flowered roses and lilies ? In spite of its infinite sadness it was enlivened by an indescribable heavenly smile. In short, I think that when nature wishes to enrich the world with new beauty she will take the lovely one as a model. The rosy lips above the teeth of ivory white seemed like fiery rubies mixed with Oriental pearls. The form of her charmingly shaped nose she had from Juno, as from Venus that of the flowery transparent cheeks. I must not forget the beauty of her slender, white, and charming neck, which certainly deserved to be adorned with precious jewels. Her jealous clothes prevented me from seeing her milk-white, finely moulded breasts. They must resemble two small, fresh, fragrant apples culled from the far-famed gardens of the Hesperides. They were so firm that through her dress one could discern their beauties and all their merits. Between them led a way at the termination of which the wanderer might expect the greatest of all bliss. The white tender hand, although it was depriving me of a part of the charming visage, compensated by its own aspect. It was long, narrow and capable, and with the most minute veins, and the delicate pretty fingers seemed to possess the power to arouse sensations even in old Priamus.

Seeing in the vicinity no one on whose account I should restrain myself, and as her kind looks inspired me with courage, I approached and said : " Madonna, if a polite question is not inconvenient to you, deign to tell me what cause retains you here so long, and if I may be granted the felicity of being of some service to you ? "

" Like you, perhaps," she replied, " I have vainly awaited the Compline of the brethren ; in regard to your offer a man of much inferior position to yours could be of service to me. My dress announces that I have been deprived of my beloved husband, and what pains me still more is that he died of the cruel plague and that on that account I am still in danger. If therefore you do not want to expose yourself to harm, remain at some distance."

The words, the voice, the manner in which she spoke, the care she seemed to entertain for my safety, all this penetrated so to my heart that for her I would have passed through fire. More from fear of displeasing her than from fear of the danger, I stopped at some short distance and enquired: "Why do you remain here so alone?"

"Because I alone have been spared."

"Do you wish to have a companion?"

"I wish for nothing more than for an honourable connexion."

"And I who until now never had any inclination to marriage, as I have seen the charm and grace of your form, on which nature has lavished all her gifts, touched by sympathy with your grief, I am resolved to choose you as my wife. Although our ages may not be suitable, yet my fortune and circumstances are such that perhaps I might render you happy."

"With you men," she said, "promises were ever great and faithfulness but small, if I call to memory some ancient stories."

I replied: "Those who write may say what they like, but he who knows how to read with intelligence only trusts those whom he may trust reasonably, and need, therefore, never rue what he has done."

But she retorted: "As heaven, the source of all that is good, has brought you to me, I cannot doubt that you will bestow loving care on me, and as you are so pleased with me it would be too great a wrong if I were not satisfied with you."

Hardly had she pronounced these words when an indolent friar—poking out his nose, who would have made a better waterman than a priest, but whose name I will suppress, so as to be the better able to express my opinion of him—darted down on this charming, gentle lady, like a hawk who has espied his prey strikes down to the earth. As if he had had a hundred intimate conversations with her, as is usual with these monks, he asked if she required his assistance. I answered him that she had already chosen a support and that his fraternal love was superfluous. The monster, who was already behaving as possessed, perhaps to procure some other connexion more in keeping with his taste, would fain have disturbed ours, as could be seen by his gleaming eyes and flattering cowl, wriggled like a snake at the magic word. But when he saw he was harshly repulsed by her, and not very kindly received by me, he wrapped himself in his cowl and took himself to the devil, mumbling in his beard I know not what.

You must not believe that I left her alone at once. On the contrary, I went maintaining a certain distance with her to her house in which she locked herself, at the same time locking herself in my heart.

When now after such an agreeable and entertaining conversation I was alone, I hastened, so as not to deviate from the order of the day which I had determined, my pace and partook myself to the excellent, cheerful church of St. Lorenzo, where I was wont to see those who had enjoyed with me the bloom of my youthful years. But the new impression was so powerful that I, like those who have drunk of Lethe's stream, had forgotten every other lady, however pretty. All my thoughts were imprisoned in the black mourning weeds which every moment I believed I saw in the hands of the intrusive, hypocritical monk, and such a fit of jealousy came over me that I could neither see nor hear anything else. I therefore concluded that I was wasting my time uselessly here, and, full of desire to see my longed-for companion again, I very soon directed my steps towards home. I put an end to the tragic description of the terrible plague, and am making preparations for the joy of the coming comedy for the next morning.

That, dearest friend, is what was revealed to my eyes on May 1st. What else there is to reveal you shall hear after the wedding, for before that I can think of nothing else.

CHAPTER X

THE FLAGELLANTS

Gigantic women from Hungary—Procession of the flagellants and their scourging procedure—Christ's letter fallen from the sky—Derision of the flagellants by Swiss men-at-arms—" The evangelical lute-player "—The flagellants as persecutors of the Jews—Cola di Rienzi—The end of the movement—The Bianchi—Stories of miracles—*Stabat Mater dolorosa*—The Inquisition.

Appendix : The Flagellant Chronicle of Hugo von Reutlingen, Statutes of the Order of Flagellants.

THE pilgrimage of the flagellants from 1348 to 1350 expressed the experience of the plague, as it appeared to the masses, in its full terror and horrible grandeur. In them mediæval asceticism and modern reformatory faith are united in a most curious manner. It is unknown by whom the movement, which already in the thirteenth century, also in times of plague, had aroused the astonishment of Europe, was once more resuscitated. The astrologists found the cause of their origin in the constellation of the third hour after midnight on March 12, 1349, when the sun entered the Ram. " Gigantic women from Hungary," tradition reports, came to Germany, divested themselves publicly of their clothes, and to the singing of all kinds of curious songs beat themselves with rods and sharp scourges.

When the flagellants—they were also called cross brethren or cross bearers—entered a town, a borough, or village in a procession, their entry was accompanied by the pealing of bells, singing, and a huge crowd of people. As they always marched two abreast the procession of the numerous penitents reached farther than the eye could see. Their heads covered with a hood above which a felt-hat was worn drawn down over the eyes, they turned their looks to the earth, and their sorrowful gestures revealed the deepest repentance and contrition.

Their feet were without shoes, and each penitent bore in his right hand a large scourge of three tails. The colour of the penitents' cloaks was black, the underclothing white, the felt-hat grey. Red crosses shone on their breasts, their backs, and on their felt-hats. Purple banners of velvet and brocade adorned with pictures and crosses, as well as torches and spiral candles, were borne in front of the procession. The people, whose feelings had been most deeply wrung by the misery of the Black Death, sobbed and cried aloud at the sight of these forms covered with "blue deadly scars and congealed blood." An incessant misericordia rose to the sky. The litany (or chant) sung by the flagellants during their procession ran :

> Our journey's done in the holy name,
> Christ Himself to Jerusalem came,
> His cross He bore in His holy hand,
> Help us, Saviour of all the land.

"And when they entered the church they closed the door and divested themselves of all their clothing, except their lower clothing, and marched in procession two abreast round the churchyard singing, as is usual when going in procession to church. And each one scourged himself on both sides, striking across the shoulder with his scourge so that the blood ran down over their ankles. And as they proceeded in this manner they sang :

> Come here for penance good and well,
> Thus we escape from burning hell.
> Lucifer's a wicked wight,
> His prey he sets with pitch alight.

As a finale of their song or hymn they sang :

> Jesus was refreshed with gall
> We, therefore, on our cross now fall.

Then they knelt down and, with their arms and hands stretched out in the form of a cross, they remained lying on the ground. And each one lay in such a position that by it the nature of his sin was indicated. If he was a perjuror, he lay on one side and stretched out three fingers beyond his head ; if he was an adulterer, he lay on his stomach ; if he was a murderer, he lay on his back. Similar postures were assumed by all others according to the manner in which they had sinned. And they remained lying on the ground for as long a time as it would take to say five paternosters. Then there came two whom they had elected as masters and gave each one a blow with the scourge, saying :

By Mary's honour free from stain,
Arise and do not sin again.

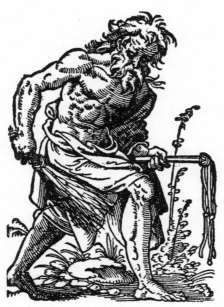

A FLAGELLANT.
From Johann Wolf's Chronicle.

He over whom the master had stepped arose and, following him, stepped across the others lying in front of him. When these two had stepped across the third, he too arose and together with them stepped across the fourth, and so on across the fifth. They copied the master in every respect, both in regard to the use of the scourge and to words. When they were all standing, the masters and the singers sang :

Your hands above your heads uplift
That God the plague may from us shift,
And now raise up your arms withal
That God's own mercy on us fall.

And then they all stretched out their arms in the form of a cross, and each one struck himself three or four blows on the breast, and all began to sing again :

> Now beat you sore
> God to adore.
> For God all pride abandon now
> And He His mercy us will show.

Then they rose up and once more proceeded, scoouring themselves so that their suffering was evident."

Heinrich of Herford describes the scourges and the procedure of scourging with the following words : " Each scourge was a kind of stick from which three

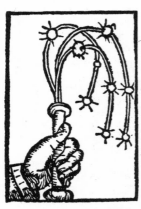

THREE-TAILED SCOURGE.
From Sebastian Muenster's "Cosmographie."

tails with large knots hung down. Right through the knots iron spikes as sharp as needles were thrust which penetrated about the length of a grain of wheat or a little more beyond the knots. With such scourges they beat themselves on their naked bodies so that they became swollen and blue, the blood ran down to the ground and bespattered the walls of the churches in which they scourged themselves. Occasionally they drove the spikes so deep into the flesh that they could only be pulled out by a second wrench." If the ceremony took place in the open it was particularly impressive when the flagellants, at the place in the hymn which refers to the passion of Christ, threw themselves down on the ground, " wherever they might be, on clean ground, on dirt, on thorns, on prickly weeds, on stinging nettled, or on stones." Hugo reports that the brethren at the termination of their scourging once more intoned the hymn " Our Journey's Done in the Holy Name," and, as at the beginning of the scourging service, formed a procession. Thereupon they marched to the cross and, bending their knees, sang the hymn " Mary, Mother and Maid " ; then again they bent their knees and their master said : " Ave Maria, sweet mother Mary ; have pity upon thy miserable Christendom." The brethren all pronounced these words after him. He further said : " Ave Maria," whereupon they all prostrated themselves in the form of a cross. Then the master ordered them to return to the passion of Christ, and once more said the words " Ave Maria." The brethren then rose up and said with him : " Comforter of all sinners, have mercy on all who have committed deadly sins." Hereupon the master again said the words " Ave Maria ! " upon which all brethren again prostrated themselves in the form of a cross. Finally, the brethren said for the third time : " Ave Maria, rose in the Kingdom of Heaven, have mercy upon us and upon all faithful souls and all that is perishable in holy Christendom." And at last the master concluded with the following exhortation : " Dear brethren, let us pray to God, that we may execute our penance and our pilgrimage so that God may preserve us from eternal damnation, and that the poor and faithful souls may be delivered from their tribulation, and that we may all gain the grace of God and all good Christians may die in this grace. Amen."

The chroniclers all report, further, that after the scourging procedure the so-called " flagellant sermon " was read. It consisted in its first part in a letter of Jesus Christ which was written by Himself on a marble tablet, which was said to have fallen from the sky on to the altar of St. Peter at Jerusalem. The letter, which actually originated in the early part of the thirteenth century, runs :

" O ye children of men, ye of little faith, ye have not believed My words : Heaven and earth will pass away, but My Word will not pass away ; ye have not repented of your sins nor kept My holy Sunday. I gave you corn and wine, and on account of your sins once more took them away. Therefore did I send against you the Saracens and heathen people, who have spilt your blood and led you into bondage. Further, I have sent tribulation upon you, earthquake, famine, beasts ; serpents, mice, and locusts ; hail, lightning and thunder, and severe disease ; but ye closed your ears and would not hearken to My voice that was in them. Then I have anew sent a great tribulation upon you, and the most evil beasts that have devoured your sons, danger of water and floods which have devastated your land, and again evil peoples who have spilt

your blood and led many of you into captivity and many
other plagues with suffering and wailing ; ye have had to eat
the dried bark of trees, all on account of your sins in regard to
the holy Sunday.   Therefore I thought to exterminate you
from the earth, ye miserable wretches; ye say that ye are
brethren, but ye are enemies—ye form family bonds, but ye do
not keep them.   Therefore I thought to exterminate you
from the earth, but My host of angels, falling at My feet,
besought Me to turn away My wrath, and I have shown
mercy.   O ye race of vipers, ye degenerate, unbelieving
generation, tremble.   Through Moses I gave unto the Jews
the law, and they did not keep it, unto you I gave baptism,
and ye did not keep it, nor My Commandments, nor holy
Sunday, the day of My resurrection, nor the feasts of My
Saints.   I swear to you by My raised right hand, if ye are not
converted and observe My Commandments, My wrath will be
vented on you, wild animals and many other beasts shall
devour you and your children, and ye shall fall beneath the
hooves of the horses of the Saracens, on account of My resurrection.   Verily, verily, I say unto you, if ye keep not My
holy Sunday from the ninth hour of the Sabbath until the
rising of the sun on Monday, and in accordance with the custom
of your fathers and brethren, holding within your hands the
cross, do not on Fridays with fasting and prayer sing litanies,
then will I pour down upon you stones glowing with fire.
Thus, I had thought to exterminate you and all living things
from the earth; but for the sake of My holy mother and for
that of the holy cherubim and seraphim who supplicate for you
both day and night, I have granted you delay.   But I swear
to you by My holy angels, if ye keep not My Sunday I will
send upon you wild beasts such as have never been seen and
wild birds, I will convert the light of the sun into darkness so
that one may slaughter the other, and there will be great
wailing and I will smother your souls with smoke, send terrible
peoples against you, who will not spare you and devastate
your land, all because ye have not kept My Sunday.   But by
My upraised hand I swear unto you, if ye do this, then My
blessing shall be granted to you, and ye shall have abundance
of all things, ye shall live in peace, no enemies shall assail you,
and at the Last Judgment ye shall receive mercy, joy, and

delight, ye shall enjoy together with My Saints in My Kingdom for eternity. Amen. But if a man should be found who should not spread this letter and report thereupon before the face of My Father, he shall be cursed, etc., etc."

The second part of the letter explained that the anger of Christ could be appeased and the plague terminated by a flagellant pilgrimage, which in accordance with the number of the years of Christ's life was to be restricted to thirty-three and a half days. The third part gives a short description of the course of the plague through a large tract of Central Europe as far as Alsace.

On the termination of the holy function the notables of the town came and invited the flagellants to a meal and a night's lodging, " and some invited twenty, some ten, each according to his means." Everywhere the flagellants were received with great hospitality and respect. Their behaviour was pious and exemplary. In accordance with their statutes they avoided all intercourse with women. Neither at inns nor at table were they permitted to speak to them. If, in spite of this, they did so, they had to confess it to the master on their knees. And the master inflicted penance by scourging on the back and pronounced the absolution formula :

> By Mary's honour free from stain,
> Arise and do not sin again.

The flagellants were not allowed to accept service, and had to sleep on straw with only a small blanket. They were not allowed to purchase anything, to take a bath, to wash their heads, or have their beards shaved without special permission of the master. What gained them the particular confidence of the people was the circumstance that each one for the time of the pilgrimage was provided with his own money and was strictly forbidden to receive alms.

The first town in which the flagellants appeared in Germany, in Lent 1349, was Dresden. Then came Luebeck, Hamburg, Magdeburg, Parchim, Erfurt, Halberstadt, Bremen, Speyer, Wuerzburg, Strasbourg, Basle, Berne, Metz, Coblence, Aix-la-Chapelle, Cologne, Frankfort-on-Main, Mayence, etc. Other towns which they visited were Lille, Doornik, Troyes,

Reims, Bruges, London, Valenciennes, Deventer; also Denmark, Sweden, and Poland.

Concerning the numbers in which the flagellants appeared in individual towns accounts vary considerably.   In Thuringia there were seen in the meadows around Erfurt frequently three thousand or more ; at Guendstadt, on the occasion of the fair, more than six thousand.   At Aix-la-Chapelle their number was so great that Emperor Charles on his way to his coronation was unable to enter the town, and was obliged to wait at Bonn till the host of flagellants had evacuated the town.   When on June 16, 1349, the flagellants went to Constance they announced that there were forty-two thousand men in their company.   A French chronicler reports that at Christmas 1349 in Hainault and Brabant more than eighty thousand flagellants had been on the march.

Derisive comments on the flagellant movement are transmitted to us only in Swiss history : " When at Berne the plague was so virulent that daily about a hundred and twenty people were buried, the Government of Berne determined to occupy the unemployed, to cheer the downhearted, and at the same time to assure the success of their political aims.   They called up the young levy of men-at-arms and dispatched them in the middle of the winter of 1350 against the nobles of the Simmen Valley, who were breaking the peace of the country and turning the highlanders from their alliance with the town.   After reunion with the contingents from Thun and Frutingen they advanced into the upper Simmen Valley. Here St. Stephen's day was being celebrated.   All the people had come down from the mountains for divine service when the Bernese army halted.   The commander ordered the pipers and drummers to play a dance, the women and girls were not coy, and soon more than a thousand armed men were seen whirling round in dance.   While singing and dancing they derided the pessimistic flagellants, who by convulsive gestures put themselves in a visionary trance and would permit of no other song but the flagellant chant.   A verse of which ran :

> To gain redemption we must pray,
> With penance all our sins repay,
> Our souls' salvation thus we gain,
> Through God's help wipe away the stain.

Instead of the ' repay ' the young Bernese substituted
' take ' and sang the following parody :

> To gain redemption we must take
> Of horse and cattle booty make ;
> Of cackling geese and fatted swine,
> We thus gain payment for our wine.

From whom the horses and cattle were to be taken, as
redemption was quite clear, as the highlanders had previously
looted the wine from the Bernese.   In the midst of the dance
the commander gave a sign, and immediately the Bernese
started off to storm the mountain fortress Luebeck, which
they carried ; they penetrated higher up the valley and took
Manenberg, the other fortress of the enemy."

The extraordinary enthusiasm aroused everywhere else by
the flagellants was not only a consequence of the moving
spectacle that they offered, but was attributable particularly
to the new ideas which harmonised with the sentiments of the
times, as is clearly expressed in their services, their statutes,
and their articles of faith.   The flagellant movement, based
emphatically on the laity, must be regarded as an attempt at
self-help on the part of the people who, deeply disappointed by
the Church, in the great distress of the Black Death, for the
first time found the courage to appeal to God directly with
supplication for help and salvation, without intervention of
the clergy.   To the empty formalism and sale of indulgences
of the Church, and the immorality of its representatives, who
publicly indulged in all excesses of lasciviousness, it opposed
the bitter earnestness of repentance, which found its most
distinct expression in the act of self-scourging.   Their cult was
a cult of repentance and, as such, was intended as a direct
imitation of Christ, such as a few centuries later was taught
by Thomas à Kempis in his splendid book.   The masters of
the fraternity must without exception be laymen.   Ignoring
the power of binding and releasing, claimed exclusively by the
Church, they arrogated to themselves not only the right to
preach, but at their flagellant services granted absolution.
Before entering the fraternity married men members required
the permission of their wives.   All were under the obligation
to forgive their enemies all evil they had done to them and to

restore all goods wrongfully acquired. " When the flagellants were asked, ' Why do ye preach having received no mission, and teach what ye do not understand, as ye are not read in the Scriptures,' they replied, turning the tables, ' Who then gave you a mission, and how do ye know that ye consecrate the body of Christ or that what ye preach is the true Gospel ? ' If they were told that the Church could not err as it was guided by the Holy Ghost, then they replied that they received their instruction and mission most directly from the Lord and the Spirit of the Lord." They repudiated the doctrine of purgatory. The Virgin Mary leads souls purged by the penance of the flagellants straight into heaven. Of the Seven Sacraments of the Roman Catholic Church only Baptism and the Sacrament of the Altar are distinguished with the predicate " holy " in the heavenly letter of 1349, whereas the Sacrament of Marriage must be kept " holy." " Marriage is a pure life, it was instituted by God Himself for us ; he who defiles it is damned." The hymns of the flagellants necessarily made a particular impression on the people, as here for the first time hymns were sung by the laity of the congregation in their own language at public divine worship. Their chants were heard throughout Germany at that time, and many of them were adapted to popular songs or even served as dance music.

At the present time flagellation is known only as a sexual aberration. It would, however, as we have seen, be a grave mistake not to see something essentially different in the mediæval movement of flagellantism. The flagellants were most earnest in their efforts to imitate Christ, and desired " to suffer the same torments, martyrdom, blows, and stripes as were borne by our Most Holy and Divine Captain, Jesus Christ, at his death." " The Evangelical Lute-player," by the Spaniard Philippus Dietz, confronts us most drastically with their motives : " A dog accustomed to lick blood and meat in a butcher's shop is hard and difficult to cure of such habits, even if driven away with blows, sticks, and whips again and again he will return. Thus it is necessary at all times, if the body is to be restrained from lasciviousness and evil desires and trained to chastity and moderation, that scourge, whips, discipline and cilicia, and such like means and painful instruments, should be ready at hand and not allowed to rest, and

even then it will only be with difficulty and exertion that the
old Adam's clay will be restricted." " If immature chestnuts
are thrown into the fire or placed on glowing coals, they give
a pop and jump out. To render them more submissive, so
that they may be better roasted, there is no better way than
to bite into them, to pierce them, or to cut a bit off. Our
bodies are like green, unripe chestnuts, which, so to say,
flourish in their carnal desires and have no liking for the fire
of divine love, but jump out and resist divine obedience. So

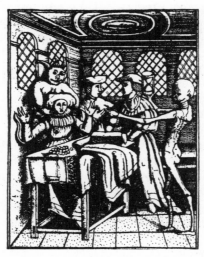

DEATH AND DEVIL FETCH A JEWISH
OLD CLOTHES DEALER.

that they may be induced to submit to reason there is no
better way than by means of the cilicia, scourge, discipline, and
such-like painful operations—so to say, bite, cut, and open
them."

The shady sides of the great pre-Reformation movement
cannot be denied. They consisted first in the spreading of the
plague by the flagellants, as they unquestionably brought the
plague to Strasbourg, and then in the fact that the flagellants
nearly everywhere participated in the agitation against the
Jews. In many towns, e.g. Frankfort-on-the-Main, it was in
the first instance due to their influence that the Jews were

burnt.   But in this they only yielded to the extraordinarily
strong popular feeling against capitalism, of which, in consequence of unfortunate circumstances, the Jews were regarded
as the chief representatives.   An old flagellant hymn says
emphatically :

> Alas ! poor profiteer,
> You sell a drachm at the price of a pound,
> But for that your soul in hell is found.

It was just in the year 1348 that the popular legend of the
return of Emperor Frederick II, " who was not dead, but
hidden away somewhere," was revived with particular intensity.   " When once he again assumed his throne," the legend
related, " then he would marry poor girls to rich men and poor
men to rich girls, grant protection to all oppressed and ill-
treated against their oppressors and procure justice for them ;
he would make the monks marry and persecute the clergy
with such vehemence that they would hastily cover up their
tonsures with anything—even if it be ox dung; he would expel
from the country the orders which had brought down the
papal bull upon him, and then with numerous armies cross the
sea, and on the Mount of Olives, or beside a dead tree, resign
the Imperial throne."

The same spirit as in this prophecy is to be found in the
message of the hermit Fra Angelo which the Ex-Tribune of
Rome, Cola di Rienzi, conveyed to King Charles in the year
1350.   Already on a previous occasion—it states among other
things—God had had the intention of destroying sinful mankind, but at the supplication of the Saints Franciscus and
Dominicus the judgment of God had been postponed till the
present time.   But as now not a single just man had survived
the Lord had, on that account, sent sore pestilence upon the
earth, and was preparing even more severe chastisement to
restore the Church to its original state of holiness.   The dawn
of a time of the Holy Spirit was imminent ; a second St. Franciscus, sent by God, would be killed by a pastor of the Church ;
but on the fourth day he would be raised from the dead, and
then, in conjunction with the elected Roman Emperor, reform
the earth universally and deprive the pastors of the Church of
their superfluity of worldly possessions.   Within a year and a

half the Pope would die and a great persecution of the clergy break out. In the place of the Pope who lived in wealth and luxury a poor Pope would be elected who, with the Emperor Charles and the Tribune, would serve as an emblem of the Holy Trinity on earth.

It is most honourable of Pope Clement VI, whom the flagellants had advised to scourge himself, and proves his great tact that in the bull which he directed against them in 1349 on October 20th he emphasised as one of their greatest crimes the persecutions of the Jews. " Already flagellants under pretence of piety have spilt the blood of Jews, which Christian charity preserves and protects, and frequently also the blood of Christians, and, when opportunity offered, they have stolen the property of the clergy and laity and have arrogated to themselves the legal authority of their superiors, on which account it is to be feared that their boldness and impudence will produce no small degree of perversion if strong steps are not immediately taken to suppress it. We therefore command our Archbishops and suffragans that in their dioceses they declare in our name as godless and forbidden all societies, meetings, uses, and statutes of the so-called flagellants, which we at the advice of our brethren have condemned, and exhort all members of such societies, the secular and monastic clergy as well as the laity, to stand aloof from the sect and never again to enter into relations with them."

It was a circumstance favourable for the Church that the King of France, the King of Rome Charles V, as well as many other authorities to whom the social political tendencies of the flagellants must be obnoxious, had requested the Pope to proceed against those heretics. Three celebrated authors had also written against the Sect of the Flagellants : Hermann de Schilde, Jean de Hagen, and Jean Gerson, Chancellor of the Church and of the University of Paris. Popular opinion was, however, so strongly in favour of the flagellants that Archbishop Baldwin of Treves " did not have his and the papal decrees announced by the parish priests, whom he would not be able to protect against the rage of the people, but entrusted them to the strong secular arms of the commandant, the sheriff, and his assistants."

Very wisely Clement in his bull had not prohibited self-scourging, but from now on everyone was to practise it in his own dwelling and under control of the Church. All who had consorted with the flagellants were obliged to do public penance at Rome during the Holy Year 1350, during which their confessors beat them on their naked backs with rods. Flagellants appeared in subsequent years in various places, as, for instance, at Muenster in the plague year 1384, but in consequence of severe persecution on the part of the Church and the authorities they were unable to maintain themselves for any length of time.

A second great movement of penance, that of the Albati or Bianchi, which broke out in consequence of the plague in 1399 in Italy, developed on more orthodox lines. This movement, according to one of the many legends, is said to have had its origin at Marseilles, according to another in England.

" Christ in the form of a Pilgrim," so the first legend relates, " appeared to a peasant in the fields and asked him for a piece of bread. The peasant regrets that he is unable to give it, as he had already eaten his bread. Christ assures him that he is mistaken, and tells him to look in his bread bag. To his great astonishment the peasant finds the bread. Christ then bids him to moisten it in the well. The peasant says that there is no well in the neighbourhood. He then goes to a place pointed out by Christ and finds a well. The mother of God is standing before it and says : ' What do you want ? ' He replies : ' I want to dip the bread in the well, a man told me to do so.' Thereupon the woman says : ' Go and tell the man that I, his mother, do not wish you to dip the bread in the well.' The peasant returns to Christ and tells him : ' Your mother, who was standing at the well, did not want me to dip the bread in the water.' Thereupon Christ said : ' My mother has always been a supplicator for sinners and is so now more than ever. But I order you, if she will not permit the whole bread to be dipped, to take one-third of it and dip it, and tell the woman that I ordered you to dip one-third in the well.' The mother of God permitted him to do this with the words : ' I see that you know this man who has come to you is my little son Christ and that I am the Virgin Mary his mother. And I tell you if I had permitted the whole of the bread to be dipped in the well the whole world would have perished, as it did once on account of the many sins of men. But now, on account of this third part of the bread, the third part of mankind will perish. But I command you to tell everything that you have seen and done to the people, so that everyone may become reconciled with God and don white clothes.' "

According to a second legend, a bull in the neighbourhood of Marseilles carried a peasant through the air to a solitary place. There, looking through the horns of the bull, he saw a angel with a book in his hand, who said to him : " Go and preach, that all should do penance and put on white clothes ; for God is angry with the race of man. And, so that all may believe you, take this book, in which is written what God intends to do with the Pope and all the people." And the peasant went to Marseilles and announced the miracle, showed the book, and related everything as the angel had ordered him. Then the bishop and the prelates began to assume white clothes, and institute processions with prayers and chants of praise.

In 1399 the Bianchi, clad in long white robes, their faces covered with veils, entered Genoa. The enthusiasm of the people was without example : " Men, women, clergy, laity, great and small, accompanied the procession ; only the nuns were not permitted to leave their convents. They marched two abreast, the women in the centre, and before each section two children. With indescribable fervour the two chanted :

> Stabat mater dolorosa
> juxta crucem lacrimosa,
> dum pendebat filius.

The whole section repeated the verse. Then the two intoned the second verse :

> Cujus animam gementem
> Contristatam et dolentem
> Pertransivit gladius.

Again the section sang ' Stabat mater dolorosa ' and repeated this verse, as often as the two intoners had finished a subsequent verse. Frequently they threw themselves on the

ground, and all shouted with a loud voice three times : ' Misericordia ! Pax ! '   Mercy, Mercy, Mercy, Peace, Peace, Peace."

The greatest miracle was that everywhere where the procession went not only the greatest emotion was seen on the
part of the spectators, but that from the moment of its
appearance all hostilities came to an end.   In places where
Guelphs and Ghibellines had opposed one another with bitter

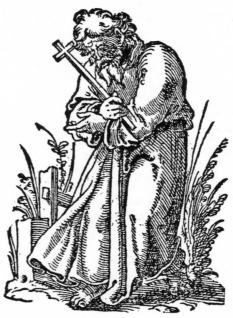

ONE OF THE ALBATI.
From Johann Wolf's Chronicle.

hostility, the enmity ceased entirely, at least for a short time.
Scholars, soldiers, merchants, burghers, peasants, all were
carried away by the same enthusiasm, among all the same
spirit of reconciliation was aroused.   Numerous miracles were
accomplished.   At the singing of the Bianchi a dead man rose
from the dead.   A man about to kill his mortal enemy
refrained, powerless on seeing the cross on his coat.   The
three months old child of the Lord of the Castle of Lerici, who
refused to conclude peace with his enemies, made the sign of

the cross and called three times " Peace and Mercy." He still hardened his heart. When the Bianchi had left his house he wanted to boil macaroni. On taking it from the fire he finds that it is full of blood. Deeply moved he assumed white clothes, made peace with everyone, and together with his whole family joined the procession.

Ultimately the Bianchi movement was also prohibited by the Pope. One of its leaders, who claimed to be John the Baptist, is said to have gone to Rome and called upon Pope Bonifaccio to renounce his dignity. Subsequently it became known that this messenger of Christ was a Jew addicted to diabolical arts, and by order of the Pope he was publicly burnt. Another leader of the Bianchi who schemed to wage war on the Pope from Lombardy and to gain possession of the Holy Chair for himself also ended at the stake. In Germany the crypto-flagellants had gained most adherents in Thuringia. They were persecuted with merciless severity and the most terrible punishments were inflicted on them. The Dominican Heinrich Schoenfeld was at that time at the head of the inquisition. From the cross-examination of those accused it was revealed that among other things they taught the following doctrines : 1. That as Christ on account of the wickedness of the priests with their buying and selling had thrown the Jewish priests out of the temple and abolished them, so on account of the lascivious priests he had condemned and abolished the Roman priesthood. 2. Since the rising of the flagellants no one could become a Christian unless he scourged himself and baptised himself in his own blood. 3. It is better that a man should die with well tanned and scourged skin than if the priests were to anoint him with a whole pound of oil.

APPENDIX

THE FLAGELLANT CHRONICLE OF HUGO VON REUTLINGEN STATUTES OF THE FLAGELLANTS

The Chronicle of Hugo von Reutlingen (1285-1360) *of the Flagellant Movement of the Year* 1349.

Let me relate to you in proper detail what happened on the earth then, in those ever memorable days, although the events and the times of which I write are doubtless known to you. At that time the flagellants were wandering about the country in crowds on all the roads and paths, cruelly martyrising their bodies themselves with blows of the cruel knots which they had tied in their scourges, for in every scourge the knots were tied threefold ; such was the order. All who joined the movement placed themselves under the sign of the cross, because all are acceptable to the Virgin's Son who without feign piously make the sign of the cross, as prescribed by the Scriptures or those who wear it. You would see a few crosses sewn on the cloaks, in the same way the brethren must provide, too, for the hats they wore. Cloaks and overclothing of this kind were worn by all of them, but their underclothing was not marked with the cross. When food was brought them they covered their heads with their hats. And it must never be omitted when the scourging goes round, as also when eating, that they should have the cross before their eyes. The cross recalls the golden sceptre of Xerxes, which was held out to everyone who desired to have access to him ; no one was allowed to approach who had not received the sign; and yet, as we read in the Book of Esther, the king was kind, prone to justice, and generous. Also to be received by Christ there is need of a sign, and this sign, as the Scriptures teach, is His cross, which He desires to see. But let us return to the flagellants and their customs. Two pieces of iron, with sharpened upper end passing through the knots, beat the backs of the penitents and caused a ring of four-cornered wounds. Priest and landgrave, knight and knave, here are all companions—even the masters of different schools are in close agreement, citizens, students, vagrants, and peasants. For thirty-four days the pilgrims spend the night in different quarters, changing each night, because for this same number of years Christ walked upon earth, dwelling in many and often poor shelters. But the last day they count only as half ; each one turns his steps homewards before it is ended. But still it is counted as a full day like the others, for Christ, too, shortened His last year on earth, rising to His Eternal Kingdom, ascending to heaven. Once during the night and twice in the daytime they tortured themselves with cruel blows, while the singing of hymns sounded with astonishing cadence and, marching in a circle, they threw themselves down to the ground and in such a manner as to form a cross. This they used to do six times a day, and they remained so long as one might say a few paternosters. When they arose there was further singing and scourging, which pained them more than that which had gone before; whilst once more they wound round in a circle, as they were ordered; their feet being bare, from the navel to the ankle, they were clad with cloth of poor quality to conceal what shame demands that we should hide; but their trunks, except their heads, they had bare. Once every night each one beat himself for the space of time during which he could say seven paternosters as quickly as he could, and during the scourging he had to cover his head with his hat and also during the night. Before sitting down to a meal each had to say two paternosters, and another three when the meal was finished. But here there was no master receiving water from his servant to wash his hands, when required in a basin; but for the common use of all there stood on the ground a vessel dripping with water for the washing of hands. It was strictly forbidden to the brethren to ask for a bath at any time or to wash their heads. No one was allowed to speak to a woman, and just as little to have his beard shorn, except in special cases when the master gave permission to some brother. Nor would anyone have dared to wear freshly washed clothes before the time for changing had duly come. They were strict in their observance of Sunday; they never marched separately, but at night they occupied separate quarters— there where yesterday one slept the next day another came. Besides, they did not sleep in beds, but their bed was straw with a light cloth spread over it—but they were permitted to place a cushion under their heads. After every five days they fasted, and on fast days they scourged themselves three times, all being assembled, and threw themselves nine times on the ground, three times at each scourging.

In regard to the number of flagellants it should be observed that they were seldom found in the same number; sometimes a thousand together were assembled in the neighbourhood of some town, frequently they marched in quite a small company, or, still more frequently, they dispersed in different groups, if they had assembled in too great numbers and wished to remain welcome guests among the lay population. And although among them were many wise, sensible men, swindlers and madmen had joined their ranks, people ripe for the hangman's rope, as they were teeming with lies, and they often annoyed the clergy and their own companions who were endeavouring to spread what is good and to avoid what is bad.

Further, all who had become brethren in this scourging fraternity had to fulfil some special duties, which we do not enumerate, all for the sake of brevity. He who went to the privy had to lay aside all clothing marked with the cross, which otherwise he must always wear. No brother was admitted without confession; anyone whom he had hurt by words, to him he must give full satisfaction; if he did not do this, whatever his rank, he was regarded as spurned by Christ and still in the toils of sin. Nor was anyone permitted to enter a house, to whomsoever it might belong, till invited by the master to enter as a guest, even if he wished to buy what he considered necessary. If no one invited them to their houses, they remained outside in the fields, or they stood in the fields till someone should let them in and give them the necessities of life and a night's lodging. They appointed masters over themselves to the number of two, sometimes only one, whose orders they observed strictly in every respect. Flags covered with crosses waved in the processions of the flagellants. Two by two, as if brothers of one family, they marched to the singing of hymns like students when on their way (they all had a common goal) to the place of scourging. The sound of bells mingles solemnly with their hymns as the procession passes through the town gate accompanied by the crowd, eager either to gaze at the wounds torn by the terrible scourges or to pray to the Lord, Who suffered on the Cross, in their hearts not to continue to destroy the people by the sudden death of the plague, to grant mercy to the dead and peace to the living till at the end of their life's course they laud and praise Him in heaven on high.

It is true that in many places abuses crept in; laity, all kinds of people, united together in swarms—indeed, even women were seen, and daily the people went out to see them without reflection. Who can tell what ultimately became of this rabble ? Therefore I make no attempt; perhaps later, if God preserves my life, I may be able to narrate their fate. But now I will end and turn aside from the flagellants to whom the people still used to throng. Some bishops, princes, and lords united and issued severe commands supported by threats of hard measures; these together with snow, frost and mist, and the impending Holy Year, ultimately put an end to the wandering companies of brethren who found the means of torturing themselves so cruelly by their terrible scourging.

Their behaviour was obnoxious to the real, true clergy on account of lying legend and insipid doctrines. They even proclaimed that on a marble tablet above the altar of St. Peter at Jerusalem the true doctrine of belief was inscribed, whereas no such tablet ever existed there. The various hymns of the brethren also contained a multitude of foolish things and doctrines which might frequently be heard from them, but by many in their honest simplicity were not recognised as such. Some good there certainly was at the bottom of the fraternity; only thus is their great success and the high respect they enjoyed to be explained. Let anyone who knows more than he has read here reveal it !

Statutes of the Order of Flagellants

(1) Those entering promise : We undertake to avoid every opportunity of doing evil to others to the best of our ability, to repent of all sins of which we are conscious and to make a general confession thereof.

(2) To dispose by legal will and testament of all legally acquired possessions or to make other arrangements, to pay all debts and restore all wrongfully acquired possessions.

(3) To live in peace, to improve our lives and show restraint towards others.

(4) To stake life and limb, goods and chattels for the defence and preservation of the rights of the Holy Church, of its honour and liberty, of its faith, doctrine, and precepts.

(5) To acknowledge that we are all created from the same material ; redeemed at the same price, endowed with one talent so that we must only call one another brother, and not companion.

(6) The novice shall request of his parish priest the permission to receive the cross from his hands; he shall also obtain permission from his legitimate wife; he shall place himself under the orders of some other and for 33½ days he shall scourge himself; he is not to sit on cushions and to sleep without shirt and without feather pillows, he must observe silence, unless granted permission to speak, he may accept alms, but may not crave them from anyone, he may only accept hospitality with the permission of his host; on going in and coming out of a house he must say five paternosters and five Ave Marias.

(7) Daily every morning he is to say three paternosters and three Ave Marias, then five times more—that is five at the bending of the knee before meals, further five times after meals, finally five at night; he shall wash his hands before meals with his knees bent to the ground and only speak at table with permission.

(8) He must not swear by the Lord's passion nor make use of blasphemous words for the rest of his life to the best of his ability.

(9) He is to fast on all Passion days, taking none but Quadragesimal food as long as he lives to the best of his ability, and on Friday he is to scourge himself three times by day and by night at such intervals as may be filled by the repetition of five paternosters and five Ave Marias.

(10) If one of the brethren should fall out with another and accuse him of falsehood, but the latter deny it, the former shall be reconciled to him according to the judgment of our confessors.

(11) No brother shall bear arms nor accept war service for anyone, except for his legal lord.

(12) No one not provided with an upper garment with short sleeves or wearing his hat may either when walking, sitting, or lying lay down his cross.

(13) No member in health or sickness may resign from the fraternity without permission, nor sit down at table without such permission.

(14) No one may scourge himself to such a degree as to fall sick or even to die,

(15) He may give alms to the poor to the full extent of his capacity.

(16) No one, however rich or of however exalted a position, may refuse alms offered in the Name of God.

(17) With head, heart, and mouth he is to persevere in the laudatory endeavours, and to pray to God for the salvation of all Christendom, that He may please to cause the present plague to cease and to forgive our sins.

(18) Should he transgress any of these commandments or act contrary to them, he is to submit to the punishment, any punishment decreed according to the judgment of the superior confessors; but he who up to the termination of the flagellant pilgrimage has been found to persevere faithfully, he shall by the Grace of God enjoy the privilege of reigning gloriously with Him.

(19) Should in the course of a pilgrimage any brother die, every other brother is to scourge himself for the space of time it would take to say five paternosters three times, and five Ave Marias three times.

(20) We decree that as a lasting memorial of the suffering of Our Lord Jesus Christ each member shall hang above his bed his dress of penance and his scourge.

(21) Most particularly he must undertake the obligation to observe complete carnal abstinence, most conscientiously observe his marriage vows, and abstain from perjury.

(22) All are carefully to abstain from carnal food on Wednesday.

CHAPTER XI

CHOREOMANIA AND CHILDREN'S PILGRIMAGES

Dancing pregnant women—Clergy and concubinage—Exorcism of the devil—St. Vitus's dance—The dancing miracle at Koelbigk—Mrs. Troffaea—A Basle servant-maid—Tarantella—The Munich Scheffler dance—*Danse macabre*—Carnival procession at Florence—Jhan Gero—Children with second sight—Flagellants of the age of twelve—The Pied Piper of Hamelin—Nicholas—The Old Man of the Mountain—Pilgrimage to Mont St. Michel—" Who is afraid of the Black Man ? "—Black Peter.

CLOSELY related to the flagellants were the dancers or chorisants, a fantastic sect believed by their contemporaries to be under diabolic influence, who appeared in 1374 on the Rhine and in Flanders. Their antics were particularly remarkable at Cologne, Treves, Metz, and Liège.

The chronicler reports as follows : " In the year 1374, in summer, there happened a curious thing on the earth, and particularly in districts of Germany on the Rhine and the Moselle—it being that the people began to dance and rush about ; they formed groups of three and danced in one place for half a day, and while dancing they fell to the ground and allowed others to trample on their bodies. By this they believed that they could cure themselves of illness. And they walked from one town to another and collected money from the people, wherever they could procure any. And this was carried on to such an extent that in the town of Cologne alone more than five hundred dancers were to be found. And it was found to be a swindle, undertaken for the purpose of obtaining money, and that a number of them both women and men might be tempted to unchastity and succumb to it. And there were found at Cologne more than a hundred women and servant maids who had no husbands. And in their dancing bouts they were all with child, and when they danced they laced up their bodies closely, so as to appear more slender. Hereupon a good many masters, particularly many good physicians, said that many of those who took to dancing were affected with too full-blooded constitutions and other natural infirmities." Another contemporary, the Dutchman Radulfus de Rivo, relates that the dancers went about half-naked and wore wreaths in their hair, " and they engaged without shame in their dances, both sexes as if possessed, in churches and in houses, and while dancing they sang and invoked the names of unheard-of devils. When the dance was over the devils tormented them with violent pains in their chests, so that with terrible voices they shouted that they were dying if they were not tightly wrapped up round their bodies. From September to October their number increased to many thousands. From Germany new dancers came flocking every day and at Liège and in the neighbourhood many who up till then had been healthy in body and soul were suddenly seized by the demons, held out their hands to the dancers, and joined in the dance. Many of the people blamed the clergy, who lived in concubinage for this, saying that probably they had not baptised the children properly. About the time of the festival of All Saints there assembled in the market town of Herstal, near Liège, a number of dancers, men and women, who resolved to proceed to Liège and to massacre all the clergy. But when they arrived at Liège, and were taken by pious people to the clergy, they did them no harm, but, on the contrary, submitted to being healed by them and their devils being exorcised. Some were taken to the Lady Chapel of the Monastery of St. Lambert, where the priest Ludwig Loves put a consecrated stole on them and read them the Gospel ' In the beginning was the word.' Thus he healed ten dancers, and gained such a reputation that sufferers of this kind were brought to him from all sides. In a similar manner dancing devils were exorcised in other churches at Liège. At Aix-la-Chapelle the priest dipped a girl, whose demon up to then had resisted all exorcism, up to her mouth in holy water. According to his statement the demon had dwelt in the girl for two years, but he was forced to come out and take himself off. By such and similar spiritual means the sect of dancers, which in the course of a year had grown beyond control, was gradually reduced. The clergy of Liège at that time acquired a great reputation."

The statements made subsequently by many of the dancers were most fantastic. They had felt as if they had been immersed in a stream of blood. Others in their ecstasy saw the heavens open and the Saviour throning on high with the mother of God. The pathological abhorrence for pointed shoes displayed by the dancers was remarkable, and the sight of anything of a red colour drove them to raving madness. There were also some who could not bear the sight of anyone weeping.

A second great dancing epidemic broke out at Strasbourg in 1518 :

> To dance at Strasbourg many hundreds began,
> To dance and to hop, both woman and man,
> In the market place, in the lanes, in the street
> Day and night not a single bit did they eat,
> Until their raging was set to rest
> St. Vitus's dance they called this pest.

The chronicle of Daniel Specklin narrates : " In 1518 there began a dancing of young and old people ; they danced day and night till they fell down; in Strasbourg over a hundred could be seen dancing at the same time. Several guildhalls were allotted to them, and in the horse and corn market a platform was erected for them and people were appointed to dance with them and make music with drums and pipes, but it was all of no avail. Many of them danced themselves to death. Then they were sent to the monastery of St. Vitus on the Rock, behind Zabern, in wagons, and they were given crosses and red shoes, and Mass was said over them. On the shoes crosses were made, both underneath and above, and chrisam (consecrated oil mixed with balm) was poured over them, and they were sprinkled with holy water in the name of St. Vitus—this cured nearly all. This evil attacked many people in consequence of being cursed by others with the wish that they should have St. Vitus's dance, and much knavery was committed in this respect."

" God send you St. Vitus's dance " or " St. Vitus plague you " were at that time a very common form of curse. On account of their evil, magic effect, they were in many towns prohibited by severe punishment. The dancing miracle of Koelbigk shows that choreomania in consequence of a curse was by no means unknown in the twelfth century. In his book, " *Schimpf und Ernst* " (Joke and Truth), the Barefoot Friar Johann Paulus narrates the following story, which is also to be found in many other chroniclers : " In the time of Emperor Henry II, in the tenth year of his reign, a tragic event took place in a village in Saxony. The patron saint of the village was St. Magnus, and in the church there was a priest whose name was Rupertus. When on Christmas morning he began to sing the first Mass at midnight eighteen persons began to sing at the same time and to dance in the churchyard, women and men. One of them was called Obertus, he was the ring-leader, and they interrupted the priest at the altar and he ordered them to desist from shouting, but they would not do so. Then the priest said : ' May it please God and St. Magnus that you should dance for a whole year.' And the curse came over them and they could not stop dancing. And a daughter of the priest was one of the dancers. Her brother ran up and seized his sister by the arm and wanted to drag her away from the dance. And he pulled off her arm, but not a drop of blood did there fall to the ground. And there these eighteen people danced and sang for a whole year without eating or drinking and without sleeping, and neither rain nor snow could touch them. They danced a hole which reached up to their waists ; they did not grow weary, nor were their clothes and boots worn out. When the year was passed a bishop of Cologne came there. His name was Herebertus ; he absolved them from the curse, so that they released one another's hands and led them into the church to the altar of St. Magnus. The daughter of the priest and two other women died at once, and the others fell asleep and slept three nights and two days. Some died, and those who remained alive walked about the country with trembling heads and quivering limbs."

It may be observed here, *en passant*, that the figure of Knecht Ruprecht (the German Santa Claus) owes his name to the priest Rupertus in the Koelbigk dancing legend. The last celebrated case of choreomania is reported from Basle in the year 1615. A servant maid made herself ill by dancing a whole month and wore out the soles of her feet. " She ate and drank but little, but danced continuously till she had wasted all her strength and had to be taken to a hospital, where she was cured. But during her dancing fit the Basle authorities ordered her to be attended by two strong men clad in red with a white feather in their hats, and these were *ex officio* obliged to relieve one another in dancing with the maniac." As a curiosity I should like to mention what Paracelsus relates of a Mrs. Troffaea, who was really the first to invent the disease of choreomania. " She was subject to curious humours, was obstinate with her husband ; if he told her to do anything she did not like it. She invented an illness, danced and pretended she could not help dancing. She hopped about, jumped into the air, sang and hummed, wriggled for some time and then fell asleep. Hereupon it came about that other women followed her example, and one put the other up to it."

In Italy at the end of the fourteenth century a species of choreomania developed from the bite of a poisonous spider— the tarantula—or rather from the dread of its consequences. As in Germany St. Vitus's dance, so this illness spread in Italy by sympathy. Music had an irresistible power over sufferers from this disease. " If during the dance the clarionets and drums broke down, for these maniacs wore out the most energetic musicians, they immediately let their joyfully agitated limbs relapse, they sank sick and exhausted to the ground, and could find no other relief than in renewed dancing. On that account care was taken that the music should continue till they were quite exhausted, and it was preferred to pay a few extra musicians to relieve one another than to allow the patients to relapse in the midst of the health-restoring dance into so discomforting a malady. A no less surprising symptom was the longing of the patients for the sea. As the dancers of St. John's night in their imagination saw the heavens open and all the glory of the saints, those who were suffering from the bite of the tarantula felt themselves attracted by the endless blue surface of the sea and lost themselves in its contemplation."—" Many demanded red clothing or to wield shining swords in their hands and with these latter imitated the fights of the gladiators ; others, when taking a short rest after dancing, made holes in the earth, filled these with water and wished to grovel in them like swine ; others again demanded mirrors and sighed when they regarded their own reflection. Many resorted to graves and desert places, lay down as if dead on funeral biers, threw themselves into wells, rolled about in filth, demanded to be beaten in various parts of their bodies, and found great relief in the exertion of running ; otherwise modest maidens and matrons lost all sense of shame, sighed, howled, made indecent gestures, and uncovered obscene parts of their bodies, etc."

In times of plague in many places country dances were instituted by the community with the express aim to dispel the general depression. It was thus that the *Schefflertanz* and the *Metzgersprung* at Munich originated, as well as the plague dance at Immenstadt and the *Siebentanz* at Kreuzwertheim. The inhabitants of Wertheim are said to have danced round a pine-tree in the forest till the Black Death left their little town. Also in the neighbourhood of Basle, near Pratteln, great plague dances were held on the Witch's Mead during the times of plague, according to popular local tradition.

In France in the fifteenth century the diseases which were supposed to be prowling about as phantasms were to be scared away by the still uglier masks of the *danse macabre*. The following incident is related in regard to the first *danse macabre*: "An adventurer of the name of Maccaber, probably of Scottish origin, accompanied the English who in 1424 flooded France, came to Paris and quartered himself in a very ancient tower, which probably dated from Roman times, in the vicinity of a chapel, round which a cemetery had been established. This Maccaber, who is described as being half a skeleton, seems to have produced a great impression on the popular imagination ; and supernatural powers were attributed to him. But his reputation increased particularly when, in 1424, he instituted a pantomime, i.e. an ecclesiastic procession, which was repeated for several months—this was called afterwards Maccaber Dance (*Danse Macabre*)—or Dance of Death. An infinite number of men and women of all ages were invited to dance by a figure representing death, and the dance took place in the cemetery where its inventor had his quarters. This gruesome entertainment lasted from

August 1424 till 1425 ; the number of participants and spectators increased daily. The churches remained empty, and the English, especially the Duke of Bedford, were not the last to take part in the spectral performance. The entertainment then ceased, but was revived in 1429." The celebrated carnival procession arranged by Piero di Cosimo in the year 1433 at Florence also belongs to this category. A huge wagon drawn by oxen rumbled along, quite black and painted over with skulls and crossbones and white crosses ; upon it stood Death with his scythe, surrounded by covered graves. From time to time the procession halted, there was a dull blast of a trumpet, the graves opened, the dead arose ; they were men in black clothes on which the outline of a skeleton was painted, and sat down on the edges of the graves and sang. The song began " Dolor, piánto, e peniténzia " (" Pain, lamentation, and penitence "), and further on the following verses occurred :

> Morti siam : come vedete :
> così morti vedrem voi.
> fummo già come voi sete,
> voi sarete come noi.[1]

Before and behind the wagon there rode dead men on meagre horses each with four servants in a similar mask, who bore black torches and a large black flag with a skull and a cross. Ten similar flags closed the procession, and thus it moved along while with tremulous voices they intoned the " Miserere."

Psychologically all these *danses macabres*, dances of death and masks, as well as the choreomania, which is also called the Dance of St. John, represent a more or less violent reaction of the enormous mass of sentiments which had accumulated in the deeply impressed minds of individuals during the time of the Black Plague. The feast of St. John the Baptist, of whom it was assumed that by his intercession everyone who sprang through the smoke of the fire lighted in his honour would remain free from illness for a whole year, was probably the first incitement to this powerful outburst.

---

[1] We are dead, as you see,
Thus dead will you also be,
We were formerly as you are,
And you will be as we are.

It would be extremely interesting to trace the effects of the Black Death on the development of music. Like a powerful spring from hard rocky ground, it bursts forth in the fifteenth century and reveals all the feverish vitality, the clashing contrasts which characterise the means of expression of post plague society. On the great motet for four voices, in two parts, " *O Roche beatissime*," by the Frenchman Jhan Gero, who lived at Ferrara, Ambros writes as follows : " That this piece was composed at the time of one of the plague epidemics by which Italy was visited in the sixteenth century, under the terrifying influence of the danger prowling in the dark, is shown by its peculiar colouring, with which nothing in the whole music of that period can be compared. The harsh clang of pain, too bold and partially purposely introduced hard dissonances, the unexpected terms of harmony, display something terrifying. Perhaps Gero received his first stimulus from the litanies for the dead with their dissonances. The whole motet is a musically expressed cry of terror, and in the whole range of the ancient art no second example of so well-considered and so well-motified emphasis of the terrible, or even horrible, could be found, except perhaps the three corpses of kings in the Campo Santo at Pisa."

The excessive unrest which during the tribulations of plague time had taken possession of humanity is further revealed by the wanderings and pilgrimages of the children. At Speyer two hundred boys of twelve years are said to have made a vow and to have scourged themselves severely. Many chroniclers report on children gifted with second sight, thus on a little girl of twelve: " Who clapped her hands and said that she saw many lights rising towards heaven, she predicted for all people in the house the day and hour of their death."

A curious children's pilgrimage is reported from Erfurt in the year 1237: " Unknown to their parents more than a thousand children left the town and wandered, dancing and hopping, across the Steigerwald, to Arnstadt. Not till the next day did the parents hear of the occurrence and fetched them back on carts. No one could say who had taken them away. Many of them are said to have remained sickly afterwards, and to have suffered particularly from tremors in their limbs and even from fits."

In the year 1284, which had been preceded by a year of violent plague, the curious remarkable story of the " Pied Piper of Hamelin " took place. " There the devil in human form walked through the streets on the day of Mary Magdalane, blew his pipe and enticed many children, boys and girls, to himself, and led them through the town gate to a hill. When he arrived there, he vanished with the children, of whom there was a very large company, so that no one knew where the children had gone. This was related by a little girl who had followed from afar to her parents, and diligent enquiries were instituted by land and water, and news sent to all places to ascertain if perhaps the children had been stolen and taken away. But no one ever found out where they had gone to."

A character similar to the Pied Piper is the legendary Nicolas, who incited the German children to start off for Jerusalem and promised them that the Mediterranean would recede before their feet. Of these children, some thousands in number, also nothing more was heard. But by many contemporaries it was assumed that the " Old Man of the Mountain " had them caught by his emissaries and was using them as eunuchs in his harem. The children's pilgrimage of 1458 is shrouded in obscurity. It was instituted in honour of the archangel Michael. More than a hundred boys between the age of eight and twelve, of Hall in Swabia, wandered against the will of their parents to Mont St. Michel in Normandy. There was no possible means of restraining them, and if it was done by force they are said to have fallen ill and even to have died. The authorities, unable to prevent the pilgrimage, at least supplied them with a guide and an ass to carry their luggage. They are said to have reached the then world-famous abbey and to have made their devotions. Further information concerning them is entirely lacking.

In the spring of the year 1709, in Lower Silesia, a great religious movement broke out among the young children of five, six, up to twelve years, which caused great sensation. In all villages and towns, thus at Breslau, " the children assembled under the open sky and sang and prayed there in spite of the severe wintry cold for many weeks, three or four times a day under the leadership of a single boy and of an usher, who punished all disobedience with blows and harsh words, each time for nearly a full hour, partly for the preservation of the schools and churches, partly for protection against war and pestilence."

An interesting remnant of the ancient dramatic representation of the dance of death is a game of catch-who-catch-can, which is particularly popular in Saxony and Switzerland under the name of " Who's afraid of the black man ? " Perhaps the card game " Black Peter " (German name for " Old Maid "), which at Basle is known as the " Black Man," owes its origin to this. According to Rochholts, the catch-who-catch-can game in Switzerland is played in the following manner : A kind of round dance is engaged in, during which the rhyme " Man of Black, don't touch my back " is sung. The dancers then draw up in a row according to size, and number off. The one who happens to have the number nine is the Black Man. His range is prescribed for him by means of a stick surmounted by a black cap, stuck in the ground ; two stones or trees form the borders of his ground. Everyone whom he catches within the limits of his ground before he reaches the goal has to join him and help him to catch the rest. " Are you afraid of the Black Man ? " he taunts the players. The more daring reply " No," and venture into his territory. " What do you do when the Black Man comes ? " he asks again. " We take to our legs " the others shout. That this game is a remnant of plague and death dances is rendered more probable by the following rhyme belonging to the fourteenth century, which stands under a picture of a child being taken away from its mother by Death :

> Alas ! O dearest mother dear !
> A black man drags me away from here.
> Why wilt thou let me go from thee,
> I cannot walk, no dance for me.

CHAPTER XII

LIFE VICTORIOUS

New fashions—Outburst of God's wrath—Intoxication of life—Guillaume
de Machant—Carrying away death—Leipzig harlots—Francesco
Berni's hymn in praise of the plague—Brandenburg dance—Hungarian
Simplicissimus—Economic and intellectual consequences of the
plague—Thanksgiving services—Hymn by a Koenigsberg plague
surgeon—The Viennese ballad-singer Augustin.

ALL chroniclers report on the returning ecstasy of life after
the plague. Thus a chronicle of Limburg narrates : " After
this, when the plague, the flagellant pilgrimages, the pilgrimages to Rome, and the slaughtering of the Jews were over, the
world once more began to live and joy returned to it, and men
began to make new clothes." The new clothes, to which we
owe the modern jacket, were particularly remarkable for the
fact that coats were cut reaching only to the hips. " And the
coats about a span above the knee ; after that the coats were
made still shorter, a span below the belt." As the coats were
very tight and lined, they could no longer be put on over the
head. They were, therefore, left open and had to be buttoned
up. This new fashion was regarded by moralists and authorities as indecent, as it closed too tightly round the forms of the
body that " it served to reveal what the sense of shame
demands that we should conceal," and in all towns dress
regulations were issued. The marked contrasts in the
different parts of the costume were particularly remarkable,
each side showed different striping, straight, square and
checked, all kinds of ornaments and symbolic signs were
embroidered on the coats, even the cut of the coat differed
from one side to the other, a wide sleeve being worn on one
side and a narrow one on the other. The allegory of colour,
which already at the end of the thirteenth century showed
slight signs of development, had now become a language
comprehensible to nearly everyone, and the full-fledged dandy

had now the means of proclaiming to the world his amorous adventures by the scale of colours displayed in his dress. Women's dress also gave rise to considerable scandal. They beautified themselves with artificial hair, always an abomination to the Church. They wore low-necked blouses and their breasts laced so high " that a candlestick could actually be put on them." Round the hips the skirts were so tight that

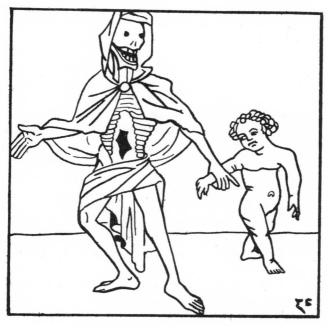

DEATH AND CHILD.
Dance of Death. German Block Book of about 1465.

with them, too, the forms indicative of sex were distinctly revealed. The pointed shoes, which had recently been condemned as one of the causes of the plague, once more came into fashion. Neither the prohibitions of the authorities nor the miracle which, according to the report of the Bohemian chronicler Benesh, God performed in 1372, was able to restrict the fashion. " As nearly all young people, prone to vanity, wore pointed shoes, Almighty God, to Whom the pride of man is repugnant, wished to show His disapproval of this vanity, and permitted that lightning coming from the sky suddenly tore oft the points from such shoes, or, so to say, the noses of the feet of a certain nobleman, Albert von Slawatin, junior, lord of the castle of Cospal near Leitmeritz, and at the same time those of his wife from both feet, leaving the persons unharmed, except that, owing to the fright, they resolved to remain no longer in that castle. But, alas! the obstinacy of mankind! Although this miracle was clearly revealed to all men, no one desisted from this vanity, but they stiffened their necks towards God and persisted in wearing short coats and pointed shoes."

The most evident cultural influence of the Black Death was the penetrating in all spheres of life and art by strongly coloured realism. In love the place of transcendental adoration of woman was assumed by a real human sensuality, allowing of warm physical sentiment. It was desired to enjoy existence to its full extent and to allow none of its transitory joys to escape. Two sterling poets, Boccaccio in his " Decamerone " and Guillaume de Machant in his " Judgment of the King of Navarre " have, independently of one another, prefaced their joyous verses, containing a full affirmation of life, by the sinister description of the plague. Like their period their poetry was by the contrast of strongly marked colours made to stand out more distinctly from the tragic background of the past.

After the plague marriages were everywhere so numerous that the priests were scarcely able to cope with the work. At Cologne after the plague of the year 1451, which carried off 21,000 people, 4,000 marriages were celebrated in the following year. Nearly all these unions were prolific and the birth of twins and triplets were more frequent than usual.

Already five years after the plague of 1348 the number of inhabitants in the majority of towns was equal to that before the epidemic. Everywhere civic life revived with surprising rapidity, and the astonishing increase of power in countries which had been devastated to such a degree as France and England once more bore testimony to the indestructibility of the human race.

The wanton joy of life which had come over humanity is also revealed in a popular song, said to have been sung in all lanes and streets in Germany :

> Ill luck all year God give to him
> Who of me made a nun,
> The black cloak on my shoulders hung
> The white skirt round my hips has strung,
> Am I against my will
> In nun's garb to appear,
> A boy's young love I yet will cheer,
> And if he brings no cheer to me,
> May that his own destruction be.

On festive occasions the people were not content with expressing their joy of life, but jeered and railed at death. From the year 1348 in many German towns the young people practised a ceremony called the expulsion of death on the first Sunday in Lent. In Leipzig this ceremony was carried out by the harlots, who at the time of the foundation of the University in the year 1409 were assembled at the Halle Gate of the town, as the so-called " fifth faculty " of the University, in their best attire, and spent the day enticing the young men. At mid-Lent they bore a straw man on a pole to the River Parthe, marching in procession two abreast and singing. Here, with a derisive song on death, the effigy was hurled into the river, and it was assumed that the town had been delivered from death. A poet of genius, of the Seicento, Francesco Berni, 1469–1536, who belonged to the genial association of " Vintners " in Rome, who made it their business to parody the most serious matters, in his poem in praise of the plague gives expression to the most unrestrained enjoyment of life. " Plague time," it says, " is the golden age, that divine first state of innocence of humanity. It is the finest time of the whole year, for then there are no talkative bores, no creditors, no crush in the churches, no schools, no boredom, no exertion, and no pecuniary troubles. It brings freedom to the individual, a wise enjoyment of life, free from all external restriction, deliberate relish of all earthy pleasures, and a turning to God and divine art."

Of the many new dances which originated after the plague, and which are closely connected with the great epidemic, I will only mention the Dance of Death, as it appeared from the fifteenth to the seventeenth century, particularly in Hungary, Silesia, and Brandenburg. It is supposed to be of Slavonic origin. " In the Dance of Death the guests paired off, young and old began to dance merrily with joyous chattering and laughter, but suddenly the music stops with a shrill note and deep silence falls upon the assembly ; shortly after a low, melancholy tune is heard which ultimately develops into a dead march, as played at funerals. A young man of the company has now to throw himself on the ground and play the dead man, the women and girls dance round him with graceful motions endeavouring to caricature mourning for the dead in as comical a manner as possible ; at the same time they sing a dirge, but sing it so merrily that it produces general laughter. On completion of the dirge the women and girls, one after another, go up to the dead man and kiss him, till finally a round dance of the whole company terminates the first part of the dance. The second part resembles the first, only that now the men and youths dance round a dead woman or girl. When now the kissing part came the fun was great, for the dancers endeavour to inflict the kiss as tenderly and comically as possible."

The " *Hungaro-Dacian Simplicissimus* " (1683) relates : " Besides in every Hungarian town I have at wakes witnessed a peculiar dance. One person lies down in the centre of the room, stretching out hands and feet, the face is covered with a handkerchief, he lies there motionless. Then the musicians are ordered to play the dance of death on the bagpipes. So soon as this begins some dancers, male and female, singing and half-crying, collect round the fellow on the floor, put his hands together on his chest, tie up his feet, turn him over on his stomach and then on his back, and play all sorts of tricks with him, even put him on his legs and dance with him. All this is horrible to see, as the fellow does not move, but stands there with stiff limbs in the position they have placed him. But I have been assured that God once punished a man for playing this part, and he who had pretended to be dead actually died and remained lying dead on the floor."

Scherer emphasises the importance of the plague for the intellectual life of the various people in the following words :

" The flagellant movement and the foundation of the first
German university (Prague, 1348) stand significantly at the
beginning of an epoch of three hundred years, reaching to the
Peace of Westphalia and comprising all religious and political
movements which prepared the way for the Reformation and
resulted from it." A detailed examination of the artistic,
literary, religious, and social forms of expression of the after-
plague period would serve to convince that the Black Death
and the preceding great epidemics of plague were not the
least active forces which contributed to the death of the
mediæval ages and to prepare the advent of modern times.

The chroniclers of strongly theological conservative tendency never ceased complaining that God's punitive judgments
had not induced to Christian humility and charity. Thus the
Florentine historian Matteo Villani expounds in a special
chapter that mankind has grown worse than formerly and the
Viennese chronicler regards the plague of 1359 as a punishment
of God, because people had forgotten the former epidemic and
had become too lascivious.

The great economic importance, above all, of the three
epidemics between 1348 and 1369 could only be satisfactorily
treated in a special treatise. Here it can only be mentioned
that the poor peasants endeavoured to avail themselves of the
favourable condition in the labour market which was due to
the tremendous loss of human life, by forming co-operative
societies, and that this led to intense unrest and great risings
of a social nature.

As at all times the large numbers of new rich were most
repulsive, spending the wealth that had come to them over
night in gross and loud pleasures and external display. The
wives of the artisans and the servant girls, Villani relates,
acquired the most beautiful and costly clothes of the wives of
rich burghers who had died of the plague and strutted about
complacently like Patrician ladies. Never before had such a
display of magnificence been seen, such richly adorned clothes,
and so much luxuriant feasting.

On the termination of the plague solemn thanksgiving
services with "Te Deums" were held in nearly all towns of
Europe. At Duelmen in Westphalia the cessation of the
plague is still commemorated every year in Easter week by a

procession of the citizens who with the burgomaster at their head, but unaccompanied by clergy, march through the brightly illuminated streets at three o'clock in the morning. The celebration at Vienna, where the memorial sermon was preached by Abraham a Santa-Clara, was particularly impressive; the preacher asked : " Where hast thou been, thou world-famed Imperial Residence in the year of our Lord Jesus Christ 1679 ? " From the sixteenth century memorial coins and plague dollars were frequently struck and issued. Thus a coin struck at Vienna in the year 1714 showed on one side a representation of the town of Vienna with superscription " *Wien ohne W(eh)* " (" Vienna without woe ") and the following rococo lines :

> Vienna now without her woe appears,
> God gives us wine of joy and wipes away our tears.
> God grant that town and State may prosper evermo'
> And, as upon this coin, Vienna be without woe.

The reverse bore the inscription :

> God by our Emperor stood, as he his friends supported
> The plague Vienna left, the best is now reported.

The state of mind of the middle class after the cessation of the plague in the eighteenth century is revealed in a touching manner by the rough verses of the Koenigsberg plague surgeon, George Emmerich :

Of patients free the plague house stands, all praise to God on high,
In our whole parish hardly now one or two old ones die,
The clerk in mournful words his burial fees deplores,
The poor give him no trade, the rich keep closed their doors.
" A glass of beer as morning drink to me is very dear,
But without corpse there's little chance for me to have such cheer."
The priest withal has little cause for grateful recognition,
Those that were sick have now begun to think of copulation.
Marcoly burns with love for Nuckel, his betrothed
Grandfather of the plague with Busch his bond has closed.
Clerk Fabian too with Morgen's Gretchen's married,
A bloodless death they would have sought, if by resistance harried.
All now are very eager our losses to repair
And to make good the dead each undertakes his share.
A new life now sets in, all praise to God in heaven,
And each himself now seeks a warm and cosy haven.

Just after coronation things to improve began,
For meat and beer our patients' mouths then ran.
Thank God that now we may enjoy a little pleasure,
Now that the mourning's done, our hearts from grief have leisure.
Till now we all a moanful wail sent upward to the sky,
And Danzic joined us in our grief with songs of misery.
But now to Thee, O Lord above, our thanks we humbly bring,
And at thanksgiving services "Hallelujah" we sing.

It can easily be imagined that the good burghers for-gathered to exchange experiences of plague time and how they particularly discussed comical incidents and miraculous escapes! Of nearly every epidemic the story is preserved of some humorous fool whom the corpse-bearers on account of his stark drunkenness mistook for a corpse and threw into the pit, where he slept off his intoxication and was the next morning pulled out none the worse for his adventure. There is a story of a merry fellow of this description, of the arch rogue Schuch of the year 1517 from Erfurt and of a Polish fellow from Danzic in 1549. In London it was the merry piper who has become celebrated through Daniel Defoe, and who was in the habit of popping up out of the carts with the dead and asking : " Am I dead or am I not ? " But the most amusing of all these characters is the Viennese ballad singer and bagpipe player—round whom so many legends have crystallised—Max Augustin, who in the midst of death retained his humour, but lost all his customers, and on that account yielded to the temptation of seeking comfort in drink. One evening, in the empty tap-room of the " Red Dragon," he had expressed his disgust at the bad state of business by writing the street-song " O Augustin, my dear," which has persisted to the present day, drunk deeply and started, far from sober, on his way home across St. Stephen's Square in Vienna. Between the Imperial Castle and St. Ulrich he was overcome by his intoxication and fell on the ground, and so deep a sleep came over him that he did not notice that the plague servants lifted him on the plague cart and then, together with the corpses, conveyed him to one of the pits and threw him in. " But as these pits were not filled in with earth till a whole series of them were full up in length and breadth, the above-mentioned fellow, after having spent a whole night among the dead without being aroused, woke up at last without knowing what had happened to him or how he had got there. He tried to scramble out of the pit, but was unable on account of its depth; he therefore trampled about on the corpses abusing them, shouting and asking who had put him there ? At last the plague servants came with the break of dawn to bring further corpses and helped him out, so that his night's lodging among the dead did him no harm at all." The fact is that this merry fellow survived till the 10th of October, 1705, when he was carried off one night after a drinking bout. His song still lives :

> O Augustin, my dear,
> Money and joy are gone, I fear,
> O Augustin, dear,
> All gone, I fear.
>
> Alas ! and rich Vienna e'en
> Is now as poor as Augustin.
> And sighs with him its mind within,
> All gone, poor Augustin.
>
> Every day some feast we had,
> Now the plague is sore and bad,
> Only corpses to be had,
> Oh, how sad !
>
> O Augustin, my dear,
> Lie down upon thy bier.
> Alas ! Vienna dear,
> All gone, I fear.

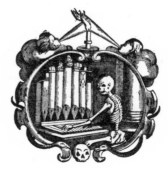

FINALE.

BIBLIOGRAPHY

ABRAHAM A SANTA-CLARA. "Merk's Wien" (Take notice, Vienna). Frankfort, 1681.
—— "Oesterreichisches Deo Gratias" (Austrian Deo Gratias). Vienna, 1680.
JOHANNES AMMIANUS. "Sonderbarer Tractat und Bericht von der Pest" (Curious Treatise and Report of the Plague). Schaffhausen, 1667.
BARTHOL. ANHORN. "Magiologia." Basle, 1675.
M. BARLACHINO. "Raggionamento sopra la peste del anno 1576" (Discussion on the plague of 1576). Firenza, 1577.
"Basel im vierzehnten Jahrhundert" (Basle in the fourteenth century), Ed. Basler historische Gesellschaft. Basle, 1856.
PETER BAYLE. "Verschiedene Gedanken bei Gelegenheit des Komet's 1680" (Various reflections on the occasion of the comet of 1680). Hamburg, 1741.
CONRAD BERTHOLD BEHRENS. "Gruendlicher Bericht von der Natur der Pest" (Thorough Report on the Nature of the Plague). Brunswick, 1714.
FRANCESCO BERNI. "Poesie burlesche" (Comic poetry). Amsterdam, 1770.
JOHANNES BINHARD. "Newe vollkommene Thuringische Chronika" (New complete Thuringian chronicle). Leipzig, 1613.
FRANZ BOEHME. "Geschichte des Tanzes in Deutschland" (History of Dancing in Germany). Leipzig, 1886.
JACQUES BOILEAU. "Histoire des Flagellants" (History of the Flagellants). Amsterdam, 1701.
T. BOUTIOT. "Études historiques" (Historical Studies). Troyes, 1857.
CASPARUS BUCHA. "Kurzer Bericht wie man sich von der Pestilenz bewahren soll" (Short treatise on how to protect oneself from the plague). Magdeburg, 1597.
ERNST BURGGRAF. "Traktat von der ungarischen Hauptschwachheit" (Treatise on the Hungarian principal disease). 1680.
J. CAPPUCINI. "Nella peste napoletana" (In the Neapolitan plague). S. Angello di Sorrento, 1884.
F. CARABELLESE. "La peste di 1348" (The plague of 1348). Rocca S. Casciano, 1897.
GIROLAMO CARDANO. "Eigene Lebensbeschreibung" (Autobiography). Jena, 1914.

PETRUS A CASTRO. " Pestis Neopolitana, Romana et Genuensis " (Neapolitan, Roman and Genoese Plague). Verona, 1657.

KASIMIR CHLEDOWSKI. " Siena." Berlin, 1923.

M. CHRISTORPHUS. " Horologium Pestis Nuntium." Hamburg, 1682.

ROLANDI CAPELLUTI CHRYSOPOLITANI. " Philosophi Parmensis." " Tractaetlein von Curier und Heylung der Pestilenzischen Beulen und Geschwehren " (Short treatise on the treatment and healing of plague boils). Frankfort-on-Main, 1640.

D. F. CLEANDER. " Was von der jetzigen Seuch der Pestilenz zu halten ist " (Thoughts on the nature of the present epidemic of plague). Berlin, 1714.

FRITSCHE CLOSENER. " Strassburger Chronik " (Strasbourg Chronicle). Stuttgart, 1843.

" Copia eines sehr klaeglichen Schreibens aus Danzig vom 22. Herbst-monat 1709 " (Copy of a most lamentable letter from Danzic of the 22nd September, 1709).

A. COPPI. " Cenni storici di alcune pestilenze," (Historical signs of some plagues). Rome, 1832.

F. CARLO DECIO. " La peste in Milano, nell' anno 1451 " (The plague at Milan in the year 1451). Milan, 1900.

DANIEL DEFOE. " The Great Plague of London."

FR. HENRI S. DENIFLE. " La désolation des églises " (The desolation of the churches). Paris, 1897–1899.

ANDREAS CHRISTIAN DIDERICH. " Historia Pestis." Hamburg, 1710.

" Die Pflicht eines Christen zur Zeit grassierender Pestilenz " (The duty of a Christian in times of plague epidemic). 1709.

PAULUS DIEZ. " Der Evangelische Lautensschlaeger " (The evan-gelical lute player). Ingolstadt, 1610.

G. TH. DITMAR. Johannes Pauli " Schimpf und Ernst " (Jesting and serious stories of Johannes Paulus). Marburg, 1856.

A. M. EGGERDES. " Neue wahrhafte Idea der Pest " (New truthful conception of the plague). Frankfort, 1715.

—— " Der grausamen Pest-Seuche gruendliche und wahrhaftige Abbildung" (Thorough and truthful description of the gruesome plague). Breslau-Liegnitz, 1720.

" Ein kurz Regiment zur Zeit der Pestilenz " (A short government in plague-time). Regensburg, no date.

" Eine wahrhaftige Ertzney und Schatz des Lebens " (A real medicine and treasure of life). Leipzig, 1517.

JAKOB FALKE. " Die deutsche Trachten und Modewelt " (German dress and fashions). Leipzig, 1858.

CLELIA FANO. " La peste bubonica a Reggio Emilia negli anni 1630–1631 " (The bubonic plague at Reggio Emilia in the years 1630–1631). Bologna, 1908.

PAUL FELGENHAUER. " Theanthropologia." 1650.

—— " Anthora, Beschreibung, was in der Zeit der Pestilenz zu gebrauchen sei " (Description of what is to be used in times of plague). Berlin, 1680.

PAUL FELGENHAUER. " Phares." 1654.
K. A. FETZER. " Der Flagellantismus als epidemische Geisteskrank-
    heit " (Flagellantism as epidemic insanity). Stuttgart, 1907.
MARSILIUS FICINUS. " Contro alla Peste " (Against plague). Florence,
    1576.
—— " De epidemiae morbo " (On infectious epidemics). 1518.
JOBUS FINCELIUS. " De Peste, Lipsiae." 1582.
—— " Wunderzeichen, wahrhaftige Beschreibung " (Signs and
    wonders, truthful description). Nuremberg, 1556.
OTTO FISCHER. " Thomas und Felix Platters und Agrippa d'Aubigny's
    Lebensbeschreibungen " (Autobiographies of Thomas and Felix
    Platter and Agrippa d'Aubigny). Munich, 1911.
HANS FOLZ. " Spruch von der Pestilenz un anfaenglich von den zeichen
    die ein kuenftige Pestilenz bedeuten " (Poem on the plague with
    introduction on signs predicting a future plague). Nuremberg, 1482.
A. A. FRARI. " Della Peste " (Concerning the plague). Venice, 1840.
PAUL FREDERIC. " De secten der Geeselaars " (Flagellant sects).
    Brussels, 1898.
PAUL GAFFAREL ET M. DE DURANTY. " La peste de 1720 à Marseille "
    (The plague of 1720 at Marseilles). Paris, 1911.
TOMMASO DEL GARBO. " Consiglio contro la pestilentia " (Advice
    against plague). Florence, 1576.
HARTMANN GRISER. " Luther, Freiburg in Breisgau." 1924.
H. GUARINONIUS. " Die Greul der Verwuestung menschlichen Gesch-
    lechts " (Atrocities of the devastation of the human race).
    Ingolstadt, 1610.
H. HAESER. " Historich-pathologische Untersuchungen" (Historic,
    pathological treatise). Dresden-Leipzig, 1893.
EVERHARD GUERNERUS HAPPEL. " Groesste Denkwuerdigkeiten der
    Welt" (The world's greatest marvels). Hamburg, 1683–1691.
J. F. C. HECKER. " Kinderfahrten" (Children's pilgrimages). Berlin,
    1845.
—— " Der schwarze Tod im 14 Jahrhundert" (The Black Death in
    the fourteenth century). Berlin, 1832.
MATTHAEUS HEMER. " Vita et gesta Sancti Sebastiani " (Life and
    achievements of St. Sebastian). Augsburg, 1702.
EUGEN HOLLAENDER. " Die Medizin in der klassichen Malerei "
    (Medicine in classical painting). Stuttgart, 1903.
ROBERT HOENIGER. " Der schwarze Tod in Deutschland " (Black
    Death in Germany). Berlin, 1882.
NICOLAUS HOEPFFNER. " Drey Goettliche Courrierer" (Three divine
    precursors). Jena, 1694.
CLÉMENT JANIN. " Les Pestes en Bourgoyne " (Plagues in Burgundy).
    Dijon, 1879.
PETRUS JURSANUS. " Lebensbeschreibung von Carolus Borromaeus "
    (Biography of Carlo Borromeo). Freiburg i. Br., 1618.
JOH. GEILER VON KAISERSPERG. " Predigten " (Sermons). Augsburg,
    1510.

ATHANASIUS KIRCHER. " Scrutinium Physico-Medicum Pestis." Leipzig, 1659.

MICHAEL KLEINLAWEL. " Strassburgische Chronik " (Strasbourg Chronicle). 1625.

ADOLPH KNIGGE. " Herrn von Antrechaus merkwuerdige Nachrichten von der Pest in Toulon " (Remarkable report of the plague at Toulon, by M. d'Antrechau). Hamburg, 1794.

LOUIS KOTELMANN. " Gesundheitspflege im Mittelalter " (Hygiene in the Mediæval Ages). Hamburg, Leipzig, 1890.

V. KRAFFT-EBING. " Zur Geschichte der Pest in Wien " (History of the plague in Vienna). Leipzig-Vienna, 1899.

JOHANN CHRISTIAN KUNDMANN. " Seltenheiten der Natur und Kunst " (Curiosities in Nature and Art). Breslau, 1737.

GOTTFRIED LAMMERT. " Geschichte der Seuchen zur Zeit des dreizigjaehrigen Krieges " (History of epidemics during the Thirty Years' War). Wiesbaden, 1890.

LANGE. " Von der Glaubwuerdigkeit der Pestberichte aus der Moldau " (Examination of the veracity of plague reports from Moldavia). Vienna, 1787.

SAM. FRIEDR. LAUTERBACH. " Fraustaedtisch Pest-Chronika " (Plague Chronicle of Fraustadt). Leipzig, 1710.

—— " Polnische Chronik " (Polish Chronicle). Frankfort-Leipzig, 1727.

ADAM VON LEBEWALDT. " Land-Stadt und Haus-Arstney Buch " (Country, town, and home book of medicine). Nuremberg, 1695.

ADAMUS A LEBEWALDT. " Chronik der merkwuerdigen Pesten " (Chronicle of remarkable plagues). Nuremberg, 1695.

JOH. FRIEDR. LE BRET. " Staatsgeschichte der Republik Venedig " (Political history of the Republic of Venice). Riga, 1769–1774.

CARL LECHER. " Das grosse Sterben in Deutschland " (The Great Plague in Germany). Innsbruck, 1884.

A. LECOY DE LA MARCHE. " Le treizième siècle littéraire et scientifique " (Literature and science in the thirteenth century). Bruges, 1894.

" Leipziger Pest-Schade und Gottesgnade " (Plague damage and God's grace at Leipzig). Altenburg, 1681.

" Limburger Chronik des Johannes, hrsg. von Rossel " (Chronicle of Limburged Rossel). Wiesbaden, 1860.

CHARLES LORMIER. " Ordonnances contre la Peste " (Remedies against the plague). Rouen, 1863.

" Luthers und Selneccers Eroterung zweier Gewissensfragen " (Luther and Selneccer's consideration on two matters of conscience). Hamburg, 1712.

GUILLAUME DE MACHANT. " Oeuvres " (Works). Paris, 1908.

ABRAH. MACHFREDUS. " Tractatus de Pestilitatibus." Liegnitz, 1618.

C. C. MAHR. " Denkschrift " (Memorial). Hamburg, 1855.

—— " Der schwarze Tod in den Herzogtuemern Sleswig und Holstein " (The Black Death in the Duchies of Schleswig and Holstein). Hamburg, 1855.

ENRICO MANDARINI. " Storia di San Rocco " (Stories of Saint Roch). Naples-Venice, 1860.

MANGET. " Traité de la peste " (Treatise on the plague). Geneva, 1721.

ALFRED MARTIN. " Geschichte der Tanzkrankheiten in Deutschland " (History of choreomania in Germany). Berlin, 1914.

A. DE MARTONNE. " La piété du moyen âge " (Piety in the Middle Ages). Paris, 1855.

CESARE MARSARI. " Saggio storico medico sulle pestilenze di Perugia " (Historical and medical essays about the plague at Perugia). Perugia, 1838.

HANS, FERD. MASSMANN. " Literatur der Totentaenze " (Bibliography of Death Dances). Leipzig, 1840.

CARL VON MAYER. " Die Pest in Bildern aus der Vergangenheit " (The plague in ancient graphic representations). St. Petersburg, 1879.

SEB. MAYR. " Ein neuer Tractat von der Pestilenz " (A new treatise on the plague). Tuebingen, 1564.

MERIAN. " Theatrum Europaeum." Frankfort-on-Main, 1637.

HEINRICH MEYER. " Pestbuechlein, aus D. M. Lutheri und D. Ludovici Rabus usw. Schriften kuertzlich verfasst " (Short treatise on the plague compiled from the writings of Dr. M. Luther and Dr. Ludovicus Rabus, etc.). Lueneburg, 1625.

JOH. C. MOEHSEN. " Beitraege zur Geschichte der Wissenschaft in der Mark Brandenburg " (Contributions to the history of Science in Mark Brandenburg). Berlin-Leipzig, 1789.

JOH. MUEHLMANN. " Geistlicher Noth-und Todesschirm, wider die schaedl. Seuche der Pestilenz " (Ecclesiastic shield from distress and death : against the harmful pestilence). S.l. 1680.

JOHANN GEORG MUELLER. " Reliquien " (Relics). Leipzig, 1803.

—— " Geschichte der Schweizer " (History of the Swiss). Tuebingen, 1810.

MURATORI. " Li tre Governi Politico, Medico, ed Ecclesiastico " (The three governments, politics, medicine, and ecclesiastics). Lucca, 1743.

ANDREAS MUSCULUS. " Gewisse und bewerte Arseney wider die Pestilenz " (Certain and tested medicine against the plague). Frankfort-on-Oder, s.a.

GUILLAUME DE NANGIS. " Chronique latine " (Latin Chronicle), Paris, 1843.

E. NICAISE. " La grande chirugie de Guy de Chauliac." Paris, 1890.

JOH. NOPP. " Aacher Chronik " (Chronicle of Aix-la-Chapelle). Cologne, 1643.

J. A. F. OZANAM. " Histoire médicale des maladies épidémiques " (Medical history of epidemic illnesses). Paris-Lyons, 1817.

J. P. PAPON. " De la peste " (On the plague). Paris, 1800.

AUREOLI THEOPHOASTI PARACELSI. " Von der Pest " (On the plague). Frankfort, 1640.

WALTER PATER. "Die Renaissance" (The Renaissance). Leipzig, 1902.

HEINO PFANNENSCHMIDT. "Zur Geschichte der deutschen und niederlaendischen Geissler" (History of the German and Dutch Flagellants). Leipzig, 1902.

L. PFEIFFER und C. ROLAND. "Pestilentia in Nummis." Tuebingen, 1882.

SIMON PISTORIS. "Ein kurz, schon und troestlich Regiment widder die schweren Krankheit der Pestilenz" (A short, good, and comforting remedy for the grievous disease of plague). Leipzig, 1506.

LOUIS PORQUET. "La peste en Normandie du XIVᵉ au XVIIᵉ siècle" (The plague in the XIVth and XVIIth centuries in Normandy). Vire, 1898.

J. A. QUERCETANUS. "Pestis Alexicacus." Leipzig, 1615.

CHRISTOPH REICHELT. "Von der schrecklichen Seuche der Pestilenz" (The terrible disease of the plague). Leipzig, 1581.

W. H. RICHTER. "Geschichte der Medizin in Russland" (History of medicine in Russia). Moscow, 1813–1817.

JOSEPHUS RIPAMONTIUS. "De Peste." Mediolani, 1641.

ALEX. RITTMANN. "Die Kulturkrankheiten der Voelker" (Cultural diseases of the nations). Bruenn, 1867.

E. L. ROCHHOLZ. "Wanderlegenden aus der oberdeutschen Pestzeit von 1348" (Wandering legends from the time of the plague of 1348 in Southern Germany). Aarau, 1887.

ROCHUS SANCTUS. "Das Leben und Legedt des heiligen Rochus" (Life and legend of St. Roch). Vienna, 1522.

PETRUS ROMMEL. "Der grausame von Gott verhengte und im Finstern schleichende Meuchel-Moerder, das ist: Gruendlicher Bericht von der Pest" (The cruel assassin decreed by God who prowled in darkness, i.e. thorough report on the plague). Frankfort, 1680.

PAUL RUNGE. "Lieder der Geissler" (Songs of the Flagellants). Leipzig, 1900.

PATRICK RUSSELL. "Treatise on the plague." 1791.

WILHELM SAHM. "Geschichte der Pest in Ostpreussen" (History of the plague in East Prussia). Leipzig, 1905.

SAMOILOWITZ. "Abhandlung ueber die Pest" (Treatise on the Plague). Leipzig, 1785.

SCHLINDLER. "Der Aberglaube des Mittelalters" (Superstition of the Middle Ages). Breslau, 1858.

C. SCHMIDT. "Kurze Lebensbeschreibung des heiligen Rochus" (Short Biography of St. Roch). Neisse, 1843.

SCHNURRER. "Chronik der Seuchen" (Chronicle of epidemics). Tuebingen, 1823.

JOH. FRIEDR. SCHREIBER. "Erfahrungen und Gedanken von der Pest in der Ukraine" (Experience and thoughts on the plague in the Ukraine). St. Petersburg, 1752.

GIOVANNI SERCAMBI. "Le croniche," (Chronicles). Rome, 1892.

HERMANN SIEBERT. "Das Tanzwunder zu Koelbigk" (The dancing miracle of Koelbigk). Leipzig, 1902.

JOSEPH ANDREAS SOHLER. "Abhandlung ueber den Veitstanz" (Treatise on St. Vitus's Dance). Vienna, 1826.

CHRISTOPH SONNTAG. "Horologium Pestis Nuntium." Hamburg, 1682.

CYRIACUS SPANGENBERG. "Historia von der flectenden Krankheit der Pestilenz" (History of the contagious disease of the plague). A.l. 1552.

GEORG STICKER. "Die Pest" (The plague). 2 vols. Giessen, 1908–1910.

ADOLF STRECKFUSS. "Berlin seit 500 Jahren" (Berlin during the last 500 years). Berlin, 1864.

HENRICUS STROMER. "Adversus pestilentiam." Leipzig, 1516.

SUSO. "Leben und Schriften" (Life and writings). Regensburg, 1829.

"Vom Leben und Sterben des heiligen Caroli Borromaei" (Life and death of St. Carlo Borromeo). Augsburg, 1611.

"Vur die Pestilenz Vil schoener Recept" (Very good prescriptions for the plague). Cologne, 1514.

Wilhelm Wachsmuth. "Europaeische Sittengeschichte" (History of European customs). Leipzig, 1831.

"Wahrhafter und eigentlicher Zustand des seligen Herrn D. Lutheri Geburtsstadt betreffend" (Truthful and actual condition of the native town of the late Dr. Luther). Eisleben, 1682.

W. WATTENBACH. "Ueber die Secte der Brueder vom freien Geiste, Sitzungsbericht der keoniglichen Preussichen Akademie der Wissenschaft" (On the sect of the fraternity of the Free Mind. Report of a meeting of the Royal Prussian Academy of Science). Berlin, 1887.

JOHANNES WEICKHMANN. "Theologischer und ausfuehrlicher Bericht von der Pestilenz" (Theological and detailed report on the plague). Zerbst, 1711.

W. R. WEITENWEBER. "Mitteilung ueber die Pest zu Prag" (Communication on the plague at Prague). Prague, 1852.

EMIL WERNNSKY. "Geschichte Kaiser Karls IV und seiner Zeit" (History of Emperor Charles IV and his times). Innsbruck, 1880–1886.

WETZER und WELTES. "Kirchenlexikon" (Church Dictionary). Freiburg i. Br., 1882–1901.

CONRAD WICKE. "Der grosse Veitstanz" (The great St. Vitus's dance). Leipzig, 1844.

"Wie man sich zu Zeiten der Pestilenz fuersehen moeg" (How to be cautious in times of plague). Vienna, 1553.

JOHANN WILLIG. "Vierzehn Predigten wider Pestilenz" (Fourteen sermons against the plague). Heidelberg, 1564.

M. DAVID WOLDER. "Historia von der groten pestilenze" (History of the great plague). Hamburg, 1506.

ERNST VON WOLZOGEN. "Hans von Schweinichens eigene Lebensbeschreibung" (Hans von Scweinichen's autobiography). Leipzig, 1885.

JACOB HEINRICH ZERNECKE. "Das verpestete Thorn" (Thorn during the plague). Thorn, 1710.

FR. G. ZIMMERMANN. "Neue Chronik von Hamburg" (New Chronicle of Hamburg). Hamburg, 1820.

GEOGRAPHICAL INDEX

INDEX OF PERSONS